The Spirulina Cookbook: Boost Your Health and Energy with Spirulina

100 Delicious and Nutritious Recipes Using Nature's Superfood

Nicholas Wood

©All rights reserved.

Disclaimer

The information contained in this eBook is meant to serve as a comprehensive collection of strategies that the author of this eBook has done research about. Summaries, strategies, tips and tricks are only recommendation by the author, and reading this eBook will not guarantee that one's results will exactly mirror the author's results. The author of the eBook has made all reasonable effort to provide current and accurate information for the readers of the eBook. The author and its associates will not be held liable for any unintentional error or omissions that may be found. The material in the eBook may include information by third parties. Third party materials comprise of opinions expressed by their owners. As such, the author of the eBook does not assume responsibility or liability for any third party material or opinions. Whether because of the progression of the internet, or the unforeseen changes in company policy and editorial submission guidelines, what is stated as fact at the time of this writing may become outdated or inapplicable later.

The eBook is copyright © 2023 with all rights reserved. It is illegal to redistribute, copy, or create derivative work from this eBook whole or in part. No parts of this report may be reproduced or retransmitted in any reproduced or retransmitted in any forms whatsoever without the writing expressed and signed permission from the author.

TABLE OF CONTENTS

TABLE OF CONTENTS..3
INTRODUCTION..8
BREAKFAST...9
1. Blue Spirulina Latte..10
2. Ocean Blue Spirulina Bowl..12
3. Blue Spirulina Pancakes...14
4. Blueberry Spirulina Overnight Oats...............................16
5. Green monster pancakes..18
6. Raw Parfait with Spirulina Milk.....................................21
7. Green Devil's Eggs..23
8. Spirulina Powder healthy Porridge................................25
9. Spirulina Breakfast Toast...27
10. Spirulina Pancakes..29
11. Spirulina Dalgona coffee..32
12. Spiral Buns...34
13. Spirulina and Chia Seed Pudding................................36
14. Spirulina and Saffron Tortillas.....................................38
15. Spirulina Milk..40
SNACKS..42
16. Aqua Blue Spirulina Coconut Bliss Balls....................43
17. Blue Spirulina Bounty Bars...45
18. Spirulina Hazelnut balls..47
19. Spirulina Popcorn...49
20. Almond Pulp Spirulina Bars...51

21. Spirulina Protein Bites..53
22. Spirulina Summer Rolls...56
23. Spirulina Cupcakes...58
24. Spirulina Glazed donuts...61
25. Spirulina Peanut Mochi..63
26. Blueberry Spirulina Muffins..65
27. Spirulina Granola Bars...68
28. Spirulina Lime Popcorn...70
29. Spirulina Almond Crescents.......................................72
MAIN COURSE..75
30. Mermaid Pasta..76
31. Corn Fish Tacos with Spirulina Blue Rice & Crema....78
32. Blue Risotto with White Fish......................................81
33. Sea Brim with Rice and Spirulina...............................83
34. Spirulina Vegetable Fried Rice....................................85
35. Spirulina Dumplings..87
SALAD..90
36. Spirulina Sea Salad...91
37. Spirulina Zucchini Noodle Salad................................94
38. Kale, Apple & Pecan Salad with Spirulina dressing.....96
39. Spirulina Spinach Salad...98
40. Spirulina Tofu Salad...100
SOUPS AND STEW...102
41. Pea soup with spirulina..103
42. Coconut Super greens & Spirulina Soup..................105
43. Spirulina Cream of Cauliflower Soup.......................108
44. Romanesco creamy soup with kale and spirulina........110

45. Pumpkin and ginger cream soup with spirulina topping 112

DESSERT 114

46. Blue Chia Pudding 115

47. Spirulina Popsicles 117

48. Coconut Blue Spirulina Raspberry Cheesecake 119

49. Spirulina Ice Cream 122

50. Healthy Spirulina Cookies 124

51. No-Bake Spirulina Cheesecake 126

52. Spirulina Meringue Baskets 129

53. Spirulina Ice Cream 131

54. Spirulina Crepe Cake 133

55. Spirulina Coconut popsicles 136

56. Blueberry Spirulina Parfait 138

57. Spirulina Pandan Cake 140

58. Spirulina Marble Bundt 142

59. Banana Spirulina Nice Cream 145

60. Spirulina and Raspberry Friands 147

61. Spirulina Truffles 150

62. Spirulina Tea Fudge 152

63. Spirulina Pumpkin Cream 154

64. Avocado Spirulina Nice Cream 156

65. Spirulina Berry Cups 158

66. Spirulina Coconut balls 160

AUCES 162

67. Spirulina Hummus 163

68. Spirulina Guacamole Dip 165

69. Spirulina Pesto..167
70. Spirulina Paté..169
71. Fresh Salsa and Spirulina..171
72. Spirulina Salad Dressing...173
SMOOTHIES AND COCKTAILS.......................................175
73. Mermaid Lemonade..176
74. Blue Smoothie Bowl...178
75. Ginger Lemonade with Blue Spirulina.........................180
76. Coconut Tequila Kefir Cocktail....................................182
77. Açai Berry Spirulina Kombucha..................................184
78. Spirulina Yogurt Smoothie...186
79. Protein Spirulina Limeade..188
80. Fruit And Cilantro Juice...190
81. Cabbage And Orange Juice..192
82. Papaya & Spirulina Smoothie......................................194
83. Blackberry Virgin paloma..196
84. Spirulina Chamomile Kefir..198
85. Spirulina Tea Latte...200
86. Green Coconut Berry Smoothie...................................202
87. Papaya & Spirulina Smoothie......................................204
88. Spirulina Avocado Smoothie..206
89. Leeks Spirulina Smoothie...208
90. Cacao Spirulina Smoothie..210
91. Spirulina shake..212
92. Spirulina & Ginger Smoothie.......................................214
93. Spirulina Limeade...216
94. Mint Chocolate Chip Shake...218

95. Vanilla Spirulina Avocado Shake..................220
96. Spirulina And Coconut Frappe..................222
97. Spirulina & Strawberry Frappé..................224
98. Spirulina Yogurt Smoothie..................226
99. Spirulina Fruit Smoothie..................228
100. Blue-green Spirulina Milk..................230
CONCLUSION..................232

INTRODUCTION

This cookbook is your ultimate guide to incorporating spirulina into your diet with ease. Spirulina is a blue-green algae that is packed with nutrients and has numerous health benefits, including boosting energy, improving digestion, and reducing inflammation. In this cookbook, you will find a wide range of recipes that use spirulina as a key ingredient, from smoothies and salads to main dishes and desserts. Whether you're a seasoned spirulina user or just starting out, this cookbook has something for everyone.

With over 50 recipes, you'll learn how to make delicious and nutritious meals that will help you feel your best. Each recipe includes detailed instructions and nutritional information, so you can easily track your intake of this superfood. Plus, the book includes information on the benefits of spirulina, how to choose and store it, and tips for incorporating it into your daily routine.

Health benefits of Spirulina:
- Lowers Cholesterol/Blood Lipids
- High In b Vitamins, Beta-Carotene, And Iron
- Can Stimulate The Production Of Antibodies
- Anti-Inflammatory
- Anti-Oxidant
- Aids In Weight Loss

BREAKFAST

1. Blue Spirulina Latte

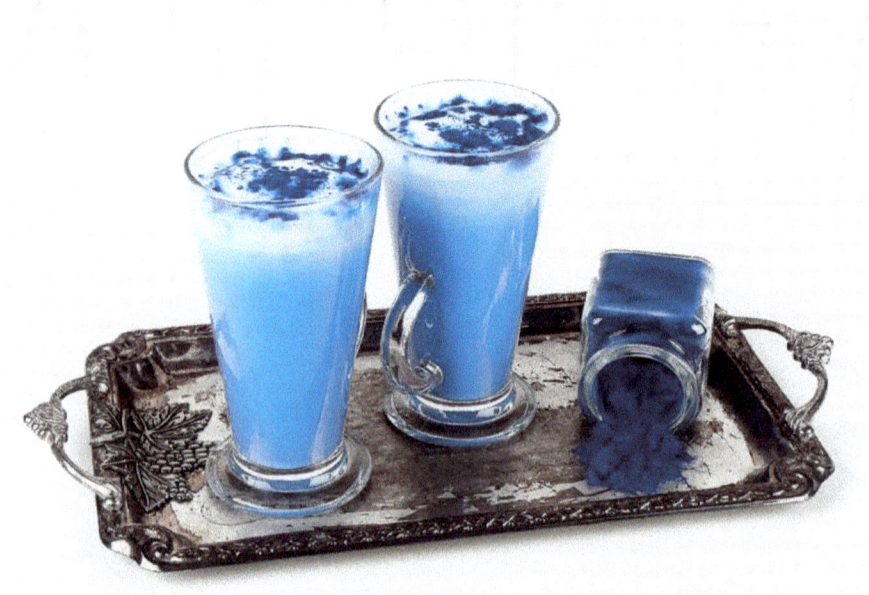

Makes: 1

INGREDIENTS:
- ½ teaspoons Blue Spirulina
- Pinch of ground cardamom
- Pinch of Ceylon cinnamon
- Pinch of ground ginger
- Bourbon vanilla
- Agave syrup to taste
- Warm almond milk
- Vegan whipped cream, to serve

INSTRUCTIONS:
a) Add the blue spirulina powder and the spices into a large mug

b) Pour a small amount of the warm almond milk over the blue spirulina powder and whisk

c) Add agave syrup and the rest of the warm frothed almond milk whisking until the powder is completely dissolved

d) Serve with vegan whipped cream!

2. Ocean Blue Spirulina Bowl

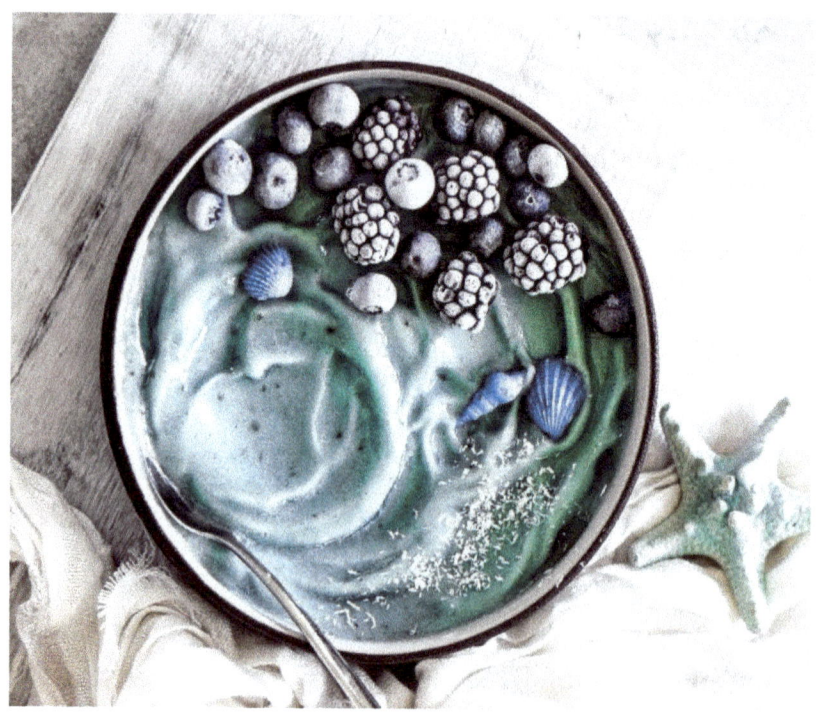

Makes: 1

INGREDIENTS:
- 2 Frozen Bananas
- a very little amount of The Organic LAB Blue Spirulina Powder
- a splash of plant-based milk
- Berries, to garnish

INSTRUCTIONS:
a) Mix all of the ingredients in a high-powered blender until they are completely smooth.

b) Garnish the top with fresh fruit and form ocean shells out of melted white chocolate using chocolate molds.

3. Blue Spirulina Pancakes

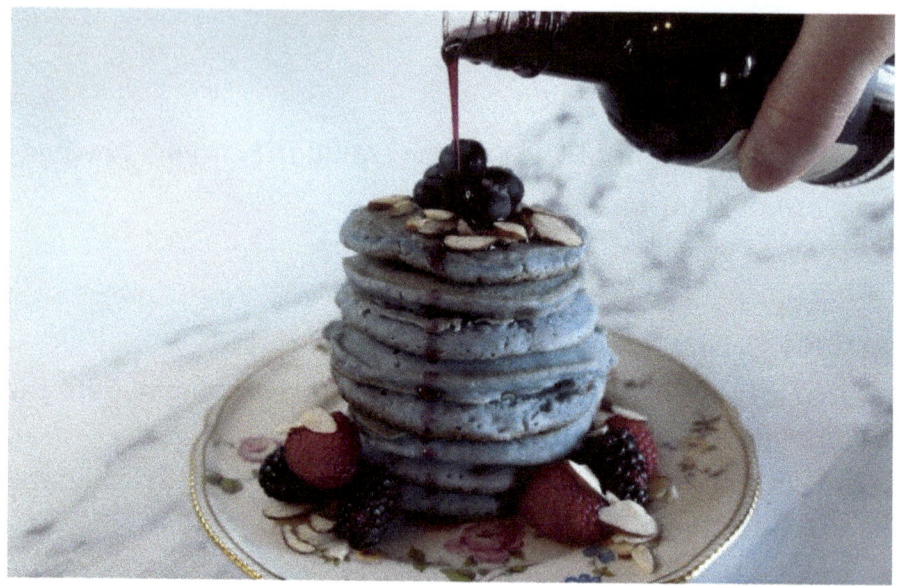

Makes: 1

INGREDIENTS:
- 100g flour
- 150ml water or almond milk
- 2 teaspoons Blue Spirulina
- ½ teaspoon organic cinnamon
- 1 teaspoon baking powder
- Stevia with vanilla
- A bit of organic coconut oil for the pan

INSTRUCTIONS:

a) Start mixing dry ingredients and then add water/almond milk and sweetener. Flip once small bubbles will show.

b) Stack your pancakes with slices of organic ripe banana in between.

c) Top with your toppings, and enjoy!

4. Blueberry Spirulina Overnight Oats

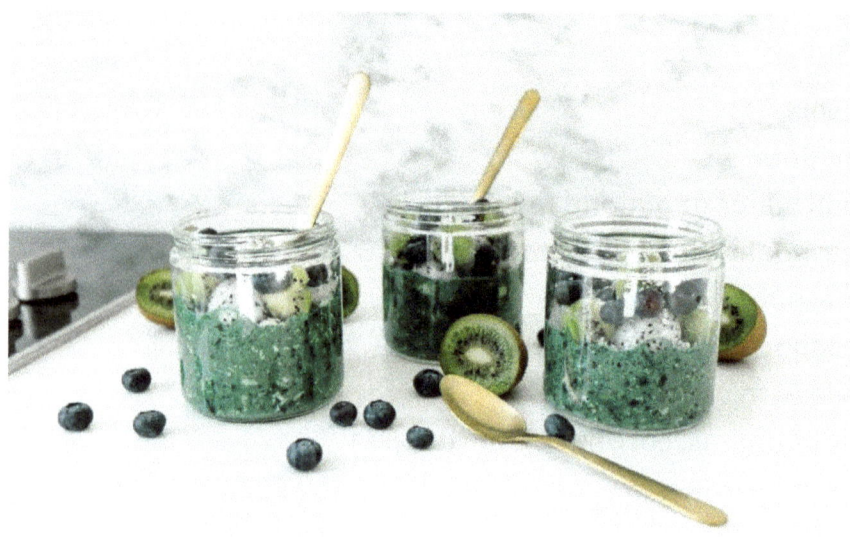

Makes: 1

INGREDIENTS:
- ½ cup oats
- 1 tablespoon shredded coconut
- ⅛ teaspoons cinnamon
- ½ teaspoons spirulina
- ½ cup plant-based milk
- 1 ½ Tablespoons plant-based yogurt
- ¼ cup frozen blueberries
- 1 teaspoon hemp seeds optional
- 1 kiwi, sliced

INSTRUCTIONS:
a) In a jar or bowl add the oats, shredded coconut, cinnamon, and spirulina.
b) Add the plant-based milk and coconut or natural yogurt.
c) Add the frozen blueberries and kiwi on top. Refrigerate overnight, or at least for an hour or more.

5. Green monster pancakes

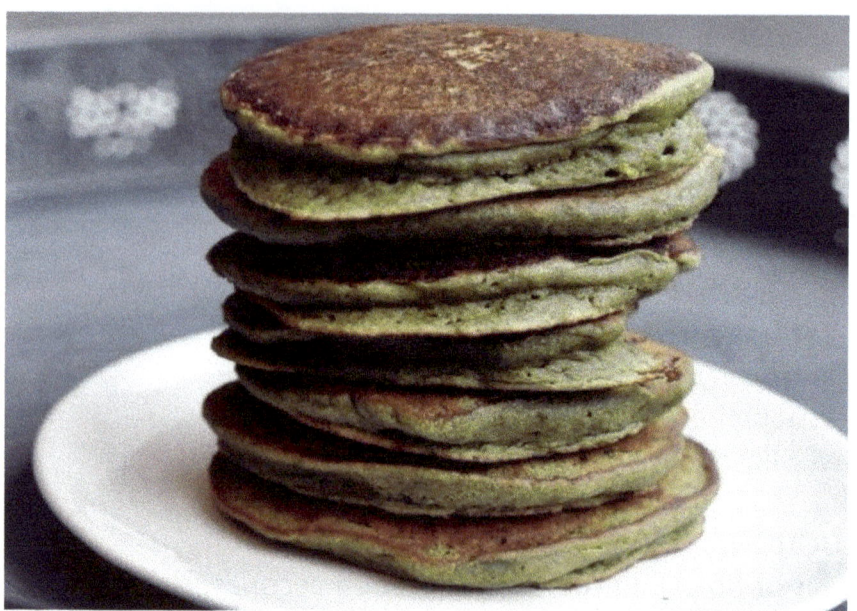

Makes: 4 Servings

INGREDIENTS:
- 1½ cups spelt flour
- 2 tablespoons hemp powder
- 1 tablespoon spirulina powder
- 1½ teaspoons baking powder
- 1 teaspoon baking soda
- ½ teaspoon salt
- 2 tablespoons coconut oil, melted
- 1½ tablespoons honey
- 1 tablespoon vanilla extract
- 2 large eggs, beaten
- ¼ cup canned full-fat coconut milk
- 1¼ cups plain kefir

INSTRUCTIONS:

a) Add the spelt flour, hemp powder, spirulina powder, baking powder, baking soda, and salt to a bowl and whisk to combine.

b) In another bowl, whisk the coconut oil, honey, vanilla, eggs, coconut milk, and kefir together until they are well combined. The melted coconut oil might harden up when combined with colder ingredients, so you can slightly warm the kefir to help prevent this from happening if you'd like.

c) Add the wet ingredients to the dry ingredients and whisk together until thoroughly combined.

d) Let the batter rest for 2 to 3 minutes. This allows all of the ingredients to come together and gives the batter a better consistency.

e) Spray a non-stick skillet or griddle generously with vegetable oil and heat over medium heat.

f) Once the skillet is hot, add the batter using a ¼-cup measuring cup and pour the batter into the skillet to make the pancake. Use the measuring cup to help shape the pancake.

g) Cook until the sides appear set and bubbles form in the middle, then flip the pancake.

h) Once the pancake is cooked on that side, remove the pancake from the heat and place it on a plate.

i) Continue these steps with the rest of the batter.

6. Raw Parfait with Spirulina Milk

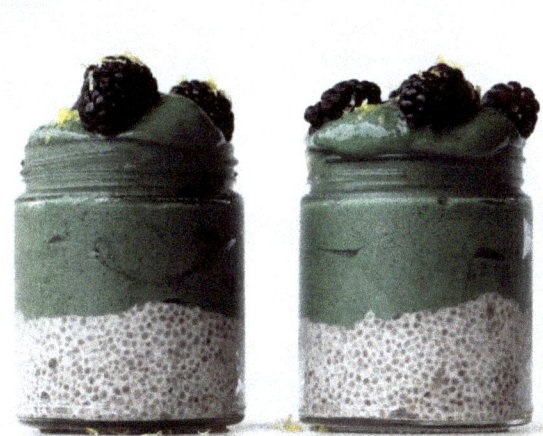

Makes: 1

INGREDIENTS:
DRY
- ½ cup oats
- 1 tablespoon apple, dried
- 1 tablespoon almonds, activated
- 1 tablespoon sweet cacao nibs
- 1 tablespoon apricots, dried, finely chopped
- ½ teaspoons vanilla powder
- 1 tablespoon maca powder

LIQUID
- 1 cup, cashew milk
- 1 tablespoon spirulina powder
- 2 Tablespoons pumpkin seeds, ground

INSTRUCTIONS:
a) In a mason jar add and layer the oats, apples, almonds, and apricots and top with cacao nibs.
b) Then place cashew milk, spirulina, and pumpkin seeds into a blender and pulse on high for one minute.
c) Pour the finished milk over the dry ingredients and enjoy.

7. Green Devil's Eggs

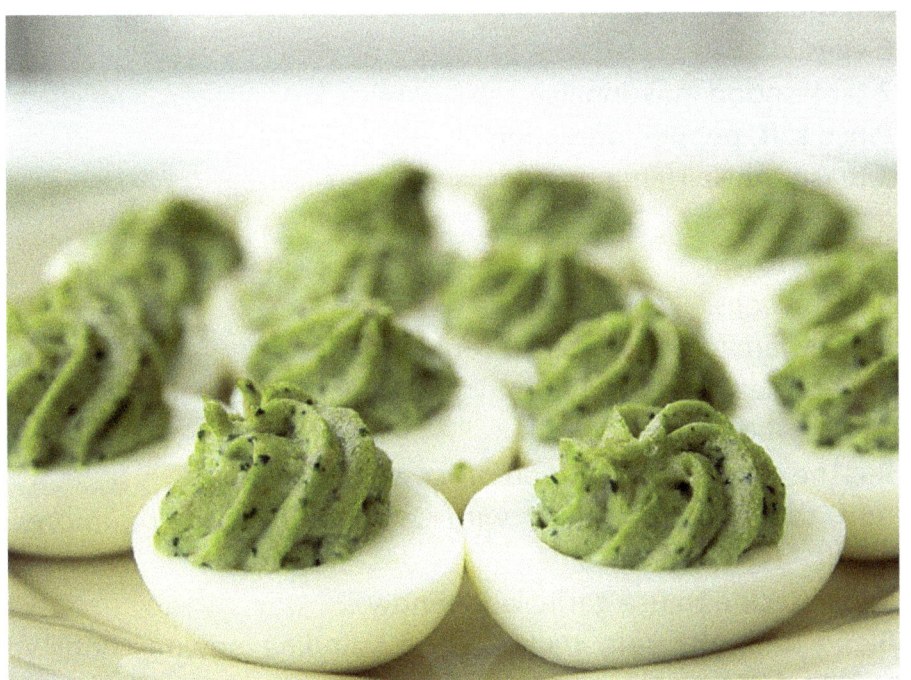

Makes: 3

INGREDIENTS:
- 6 eggs
- 2 tablespoon mayonnaise
- Pinch salt, pepper, and paprika
- 1 teaspoon spirulina powder

INSTRUCTIONS:
a) Boil the eggs.
b) Rinse them in cold water to cool them down
c) Peel the eggs and cut them in half lengthwise making sure you keep the white intact
d) Put the egg yolk into a food processor.
e) Add the mayo, starting with 2 spoonful's adding more if needed.
f) If you decide to use garlic, add it now.
g) Blend with the salt, pepper, and Spirulina powder until you have a uniform paste.
h) Scoop the yolk back into the center of the egg whites.
i) Sprinkle lightly with paprika for extra color.

8. Spirulina Powder healthy Porridge

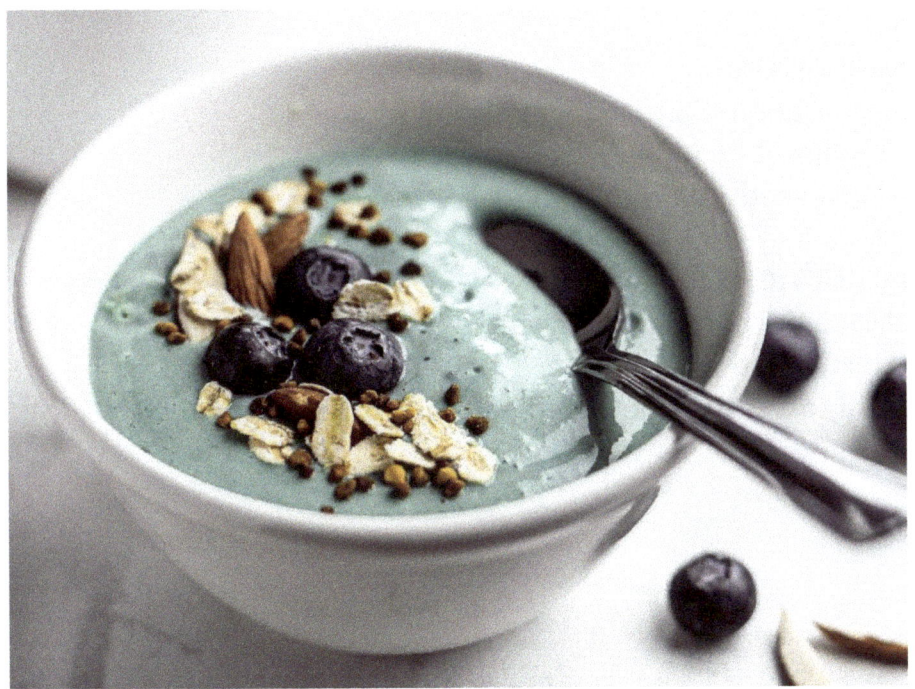

Makes: 1 serving

INGREDIENTS:
- ½ teaspoons Spirulina Powder
- 1 tablespoon Milk
- Some seeds to finish

INSTRUCTIONS:
a) Make the porridge with water and add the milk and stir.
b) Next, add the Spirulina,
c) Add to a serving bowl and add some seeds on top.

9. Spirulina Breakfast Toast

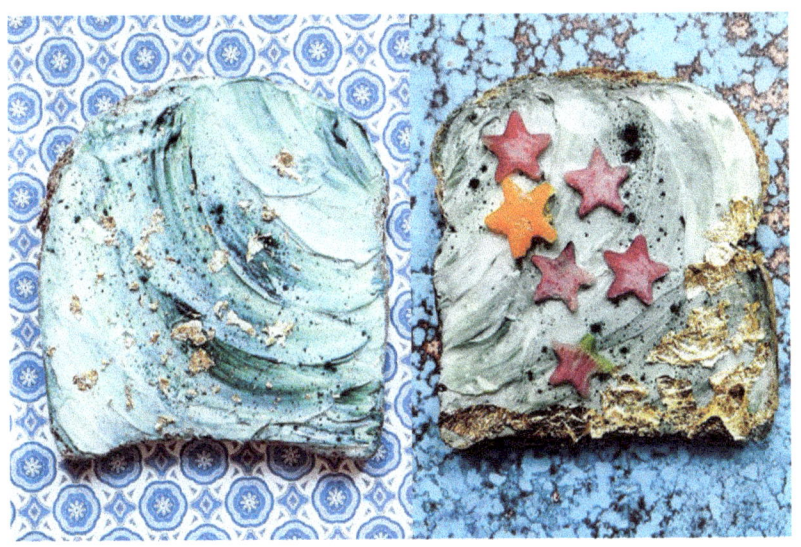

Makes: 1 serving

INGREDIENTS:
- 2 tablespoons Greek yogurt
- Lemon juice to taste
- 1 teaspoon Spirulina Powder
- Two pieces of whole-wheat bread

INSTRUCTIONS:
a) Mix Greek yogurt, lemon juice, and spirulina powder.
b) Spread onto two pieces of toast
c) Add toppings of choice. We recommend hard-boiled eggs, tuna, and avocado for an extra-filling meal.

10. Spirulina Pancakes

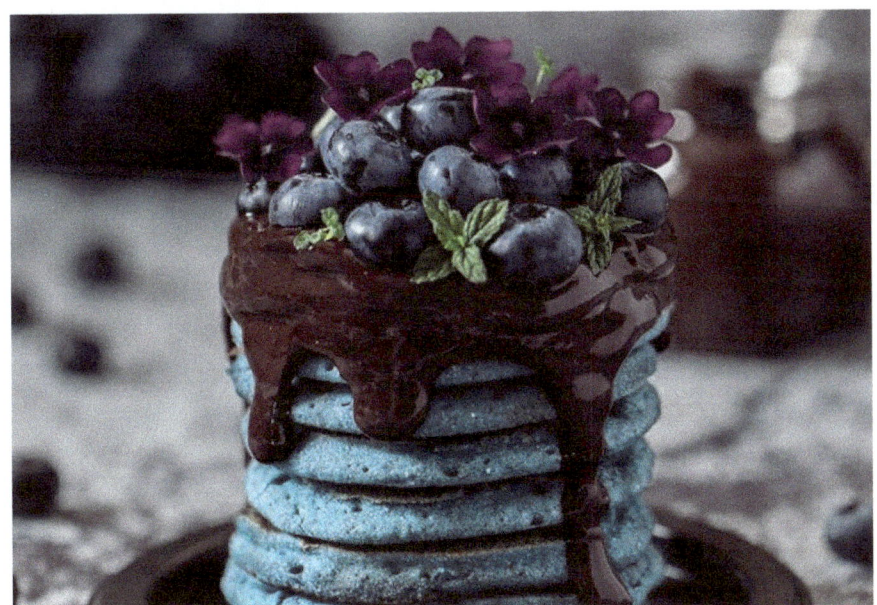

Makes: 15 pancakes

INGREDIENTS:
PANCAKES
- 80 g fine buckwheat flour
- 80 g white rice flour
- 2 teaspoons baking powder
- 2 teaspoons Spirulina powder
- 7 tablespoons agave
- 160 ml of almond milk

CHOCOLATE SAUCE
- 60 g coconut cream
- 50 g dark chocolate
- 1 tablespoon coconut oil
- 1-2 tablespoons agave

TOPPING
- Mint
- Blueberries

INSTRUCTIONS:
PANCAKES
a) Place buckwheat flour, white rice flour, Spirulina powder, and baking powder in a medium-sized bowl.
b) Add 160 ml rice milk and agave syrup, and mix briefly with a hand mixer until well combined. Adjust sweetness.
c) If the batter is too thick, add 1 extra tablespoon rice milk.
d) Brush the pan with coconut oil and preheat it under medium-low heat.
e) Pour the batter into a small circle. When the pancakes start bubbling a bit and the bottom is lightly browned, flip them over and cook briefly on the other side.

CHOCOLATE SAUCE
f) Melt chocolate with 1 tablespoon coconut oil over low heat in a medium pot. Stir until smooth. Let it cool down a bit.

g) Add coconut cream, melted chocolate, and agave to the blender and blend briefly until smooth.

h) Serve pancakes with chocolate sauce and top with blueberries and mint leaves.

11. Spirulina Dalgona coffee

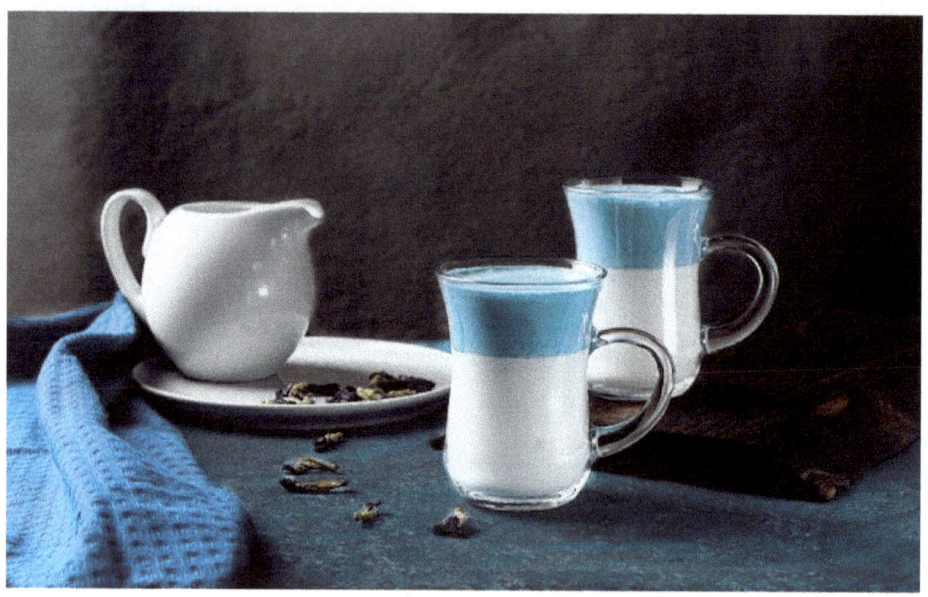

Makes: 2

INGREDIENTS:
- 2 tablespoons sugar
- 2 tablespoons boiling water
- Liquid from a can of chickpeas/aquafaba
- 1 teaspoon Spirulina powder
- 2 cups oat milk

INSTRUCTIONS:
a) Strain can of chickpeas into a bowl to use the liquid from the can.
b) Use a handheld electric mixer to whip them until fluffy.
c) Meanwhile boil water and pour two tablespoons in a bowl with sugar and Spirulina powder to dissolve. Once the aquafaba is frothy, add in the blue bowl of sugary goodness.
d) Whip until frothy! Be patient.
e) Fill two mini small jars with oat milk and ice and spoon the frothy blue on top.

12. Spiral Buns

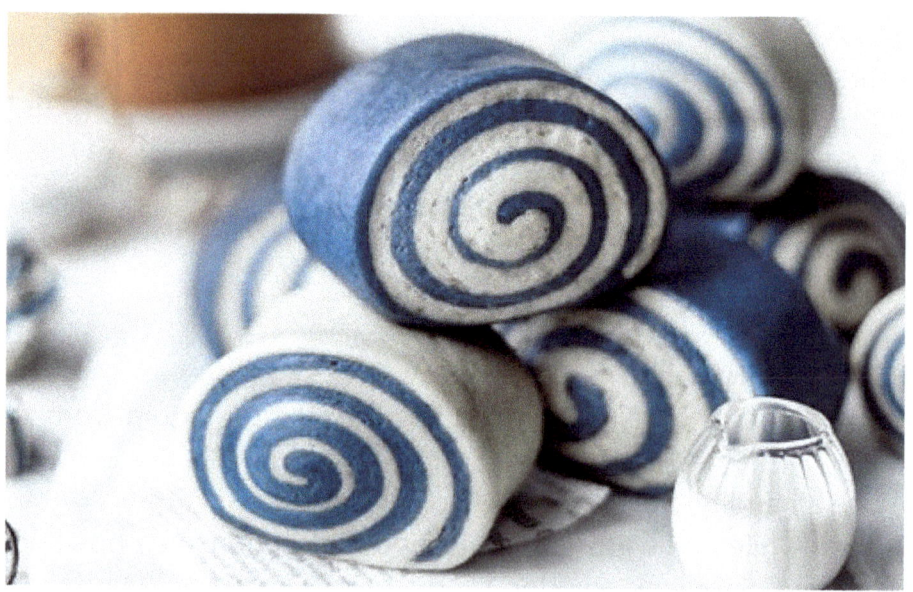

INGREDIENTS:
- 1 ½ cups all-purpose flour
- ½ teaspoon instant yeast
- 1 tablespoon sugar
- ½ cup plant-based milk
- ½ tablespoons vegetable oil

FLAVOUR & COLORING:
- 1 teaspoon Spirulina powder, dissolved in 1 teaspoon plant-based milk

INSTRUCTIONS:
a) In a large mixing bowl combine all dry ingredients, add in oil and milk gradually, mix into a dough. Cover the bowl and let the dough rest for 15 minutes.
b) Divide dough into 2. Knead the plain dough until smooth, elastic, and shiny. Cover with kitchen towel to prevent it from drying out.
c) Add the dissolved Spirulina powder mixture to the second portion of dough, knead until well incorporated, dough becomes smooth, elastic, and shiny.
d) Roll out the plain dough on parchment paper, roll out into thin flat rectangle. Set aside.
e) Roll out the Spirulina dough on parchment paper, roll out into thin flat rectangle.
f) Gently stack the blue dough on top of the plain. Use a rolling pin to seal the two layers. Gently roll the dough into a log. Cut log into about 6 equal pieces and place them on parchment paper squares. Cover and set in a warm place to rise for 20 minutes.
g) Steam buns for 15 minutes on low heat. Serve warm. Enjoy!

13. Spirulina and Chia Seed Pudding

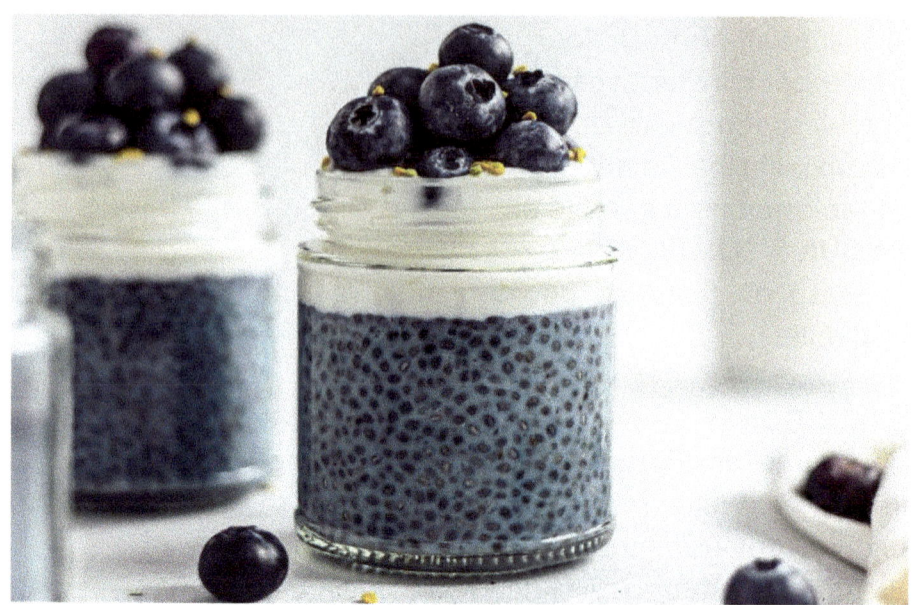

INGREDIENTS
- 2 tablespoons spirulina powder
- 1-½ cups almond milk, at 200°F
- 1 tablespoon honey or agave
- 4 tablespoons chia seeds

TO SERVE:
- 1 cup Greek yogurt
- Handful of berries

INSTRUCTIONS:
a) Add the hot almond milk to the spirulina and steep for 3-5 minutes.
b) In a container with a lid, add the sweetener and chia seeds.
c) Stir to combine and refrigerate overnight.

TO SERVE:
d) In a cup or small bowl, layer in Greek yogurt, and the two different chia puddings to create parfait layers.
e) Garnish with berries and more honey as desired. Serve cold.

14. Spirulina and Saffron Tortillas

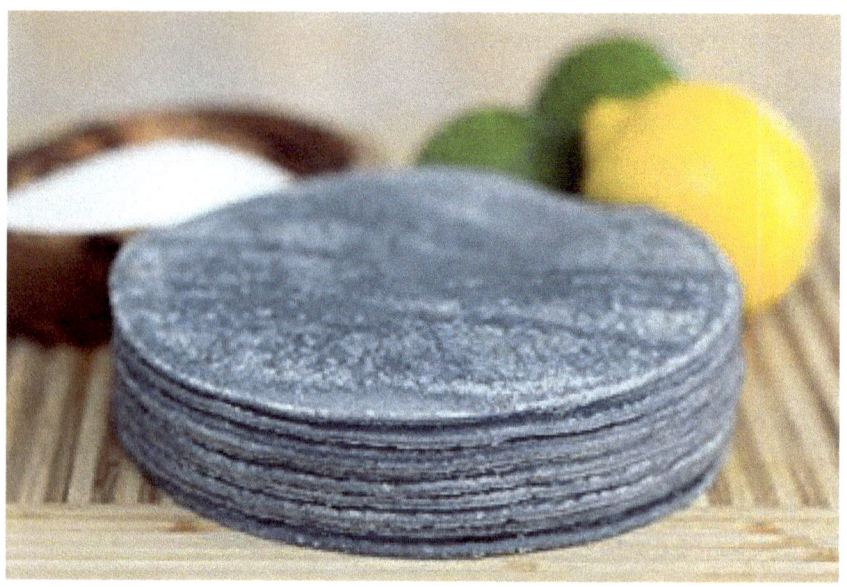

INGREDIENTS
- 2 cups unbleached all-purpose flour
- ½ teaspoon salt
- ¼ cup vegetable oil
- ⅔ cup boiling water
- 1 tablespoon of Spirulina
- 2 pinches of Saffron

INSTRUCTIONS:
a) Steep Spirulina in ⅔ cup boiling water or saffron in ⅔ cup boiling water.
b) When water cools to warm, then make the tortillas.
c) Combine flour and salt together. Add oil, and mix until the mixture resembles small peas.
d) Add the steeped warm water and mix well, scraping down the sides of the bowl. It should form into a ball.
e) Lightly flour a cutting board and knead the ball for about a minute. Then cover the dough ball and let rest for at least 30 minutes, but no more than a couple of hours.
f) Heat up a pancake griddle or a couple of Teflon pans. You want it to be medium hot. Form dough into little balls.
g) Your Makes will obviously vary depending on the size you roll.
h) Flatten a dough ball with your hands, and then place on a cutting board.
i) Roll out to the thickness you want your tortilla to be.
j) Place the rolled out tortilla on the hot pan/griddle surface and watch it cook.
k) Using a spatula, lift up the tortilla to see if it's done. It should be browned on the bottom - if it is, then it's ready to flip over and cook the other side.
l) Cook that side until brown, and remove and put on a plate to cool.
m) Repeat with the rest of your dough, continuing to stack them on top of each other when fully cooked.

15. Spirulina Milk

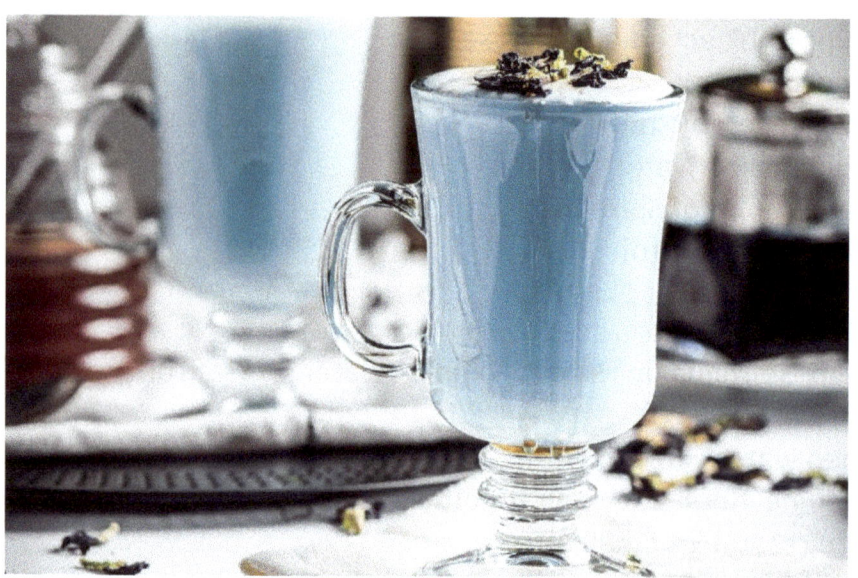

Makes: 4 servings

INGREDIENTS:
- 2 tablespoons Spirulina powder
- 2 cups filtered water
- ½ cup raw cashews
- ½ cup raw almonds
- 3 pitted dates
- ½ teaspoon vanilla extract
- pinch of sea salt

INSTRUCTIONS:
a) Soak the cashews and almonds for at least 2 hours in the water, and discard the water after soaking.
b) Blend all the ingredients in a blender until smooth. Chill before enjoying.

SNACKS

16. Aqua Blue Spirulina Coconut Bliss Balls

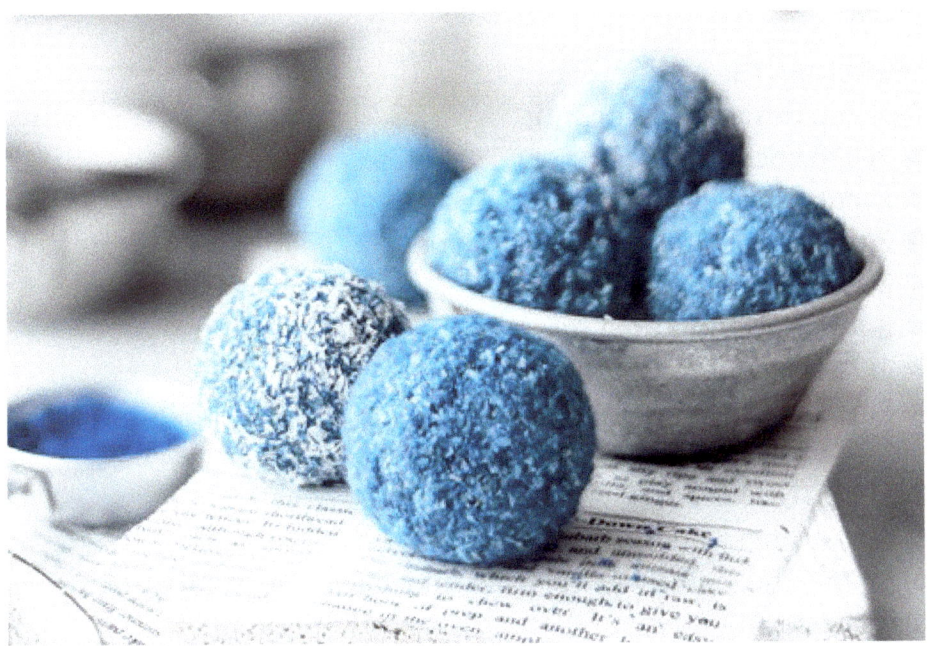

Makes: 4 servings

INGREDIENTS:
- ¾ cup desiccated Coconut
- ⅓ cup coconut flour
- ⅓ cup pitted dates, soaked
- 2 teaspoons Blue Spirulina Powder
- 3 tablespoons coconut butter
- 3 tablespoons maple syrup
- 1-2 tablespoons coconut oil
- Pinch of Salt

INSTRUCTIONS:
a) Add all ingredients into a food processor and pulse.
b) Shape the mixture into balls and place on a parchment-lined plate or baking tray.
c) Roll balls into more coconut if desired.
d) Freeze bars for at least 1-2 hours until set.

17. Blue Spirulina Bounty Bars

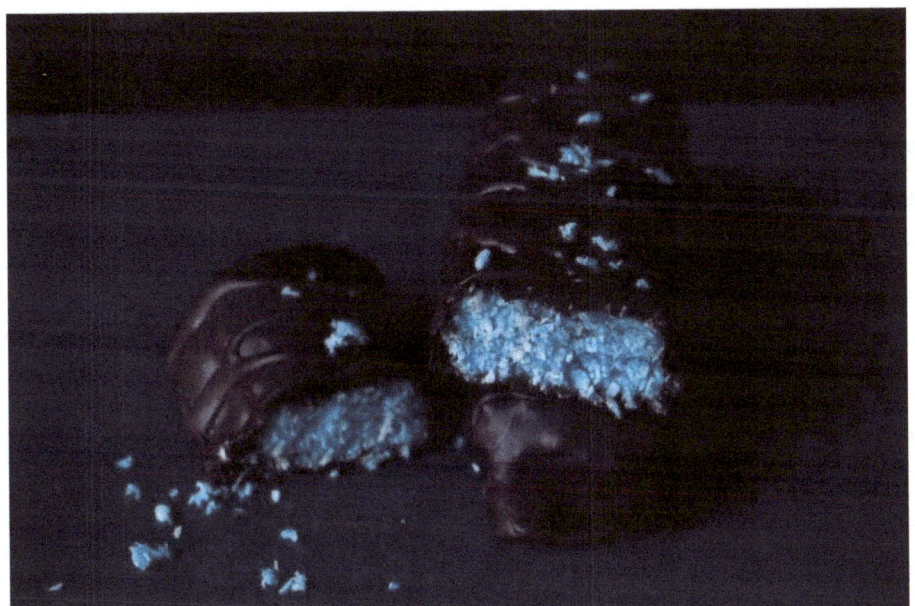

Makes: 4 servings

INGREDIENTS:
- 1 cup shredded coconut
- 3 tablespoons rice syrup
- 2 tablespoons Coconut milk
- 1 tablespoon coconut oil
- 1 teaspoon spirulina
- 1 tablespoon coconut oil
- 2.5 oz dark chocolate

INSTRUCTIONS:
a) Line a loaf pan with parchment paper or use a silicone pan

b) In a bowl, mix the unsweetened shredded coconut, the coconut milk, the rice syrup, the melted coconut oil, and the spirulina thoroughly with a spoon or use your hands as I did

c) Press the whole mixture evenly into your lined loaf pan and cut them later

d) Transfer to the freezer for about 1 hour

e) Next, melt the dark chocolate with the coconut oil

f) Use a fork placed underneath, dip every bar into the chocolate

g) Then place your chocolate-covered bars back on the carving board and transfer them back to the freezer for an additional 30 minutes.

18. Spirulina Hazelnut balls

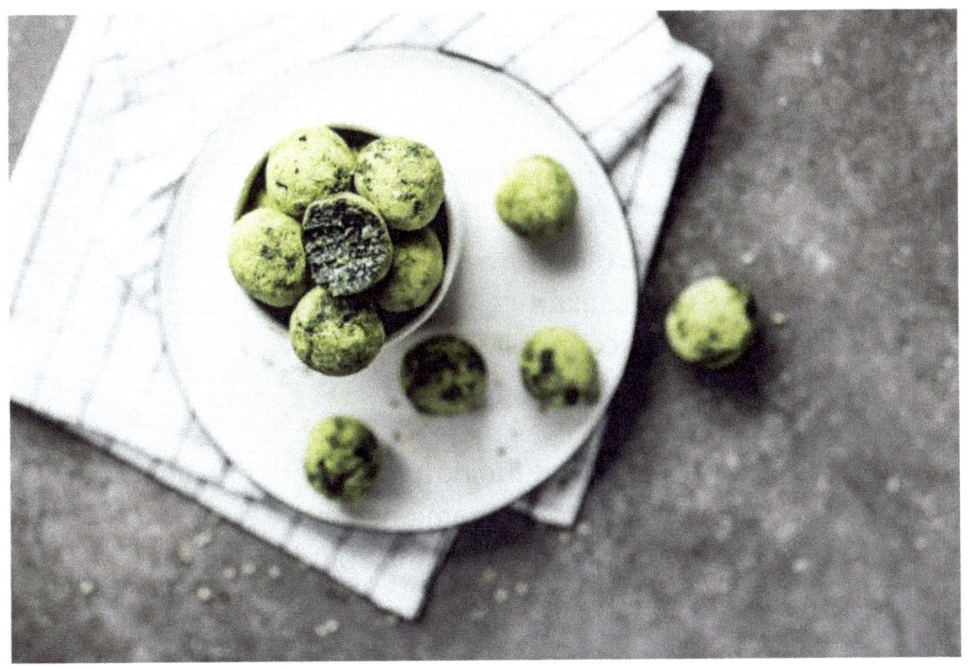

Makes: 10-15 balls

INGREDIENTS:
- grated lemon zest from 2 lemons
- 3 cups hazelnuts
- 1 tablespoon spirulina powder
- 1½ cups raisins, soaked
- 2 tablespoons coconut oil

INSTRUCTIONS:
a) In a food processor, grind the hazelnuts until finely ground.
b) Add the raisins and process them once more.
c) Add the coconut oil, lemon zest, and spirulina powder.
d) Roll into bite-sized balls.

19. Spirulina Popcorn

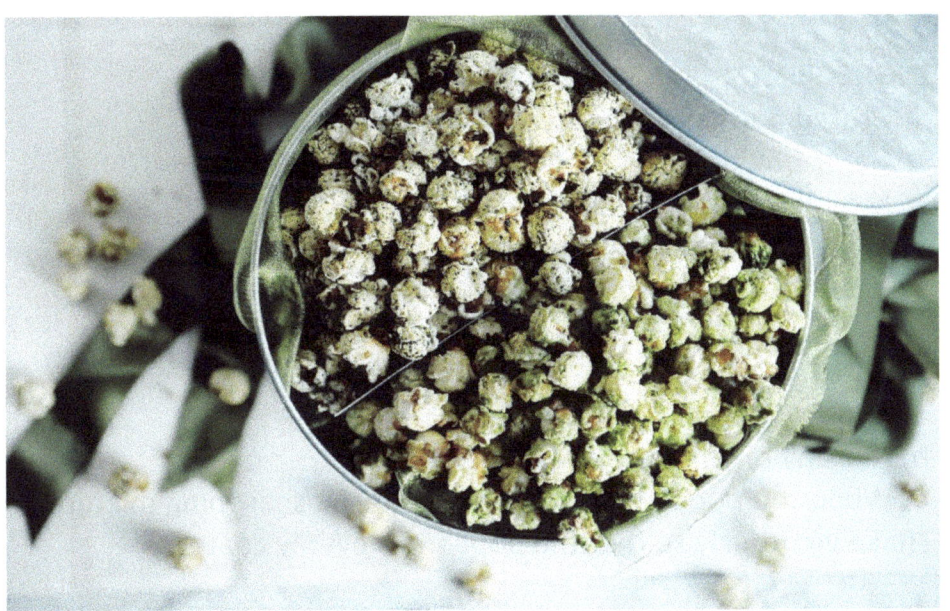

Makes: 4 servings

INGREDIENTS:
- Grated parmesan cheese
- Garlic powder
- ½ tablespoon dulse flakes
- Cayenne pepper, chili pepper, or paprika
- 1 tablespoon Spirulina

INSTRUCTIONS:
a) Make popcorn as usual.
b) Mix any or all of the above ingredients.
c) While the popcorn is still warm, add the seasoning mixture and shake vigorously so that the popcorn is evenly coated.

20. Almond Pulp Spirulina Bars

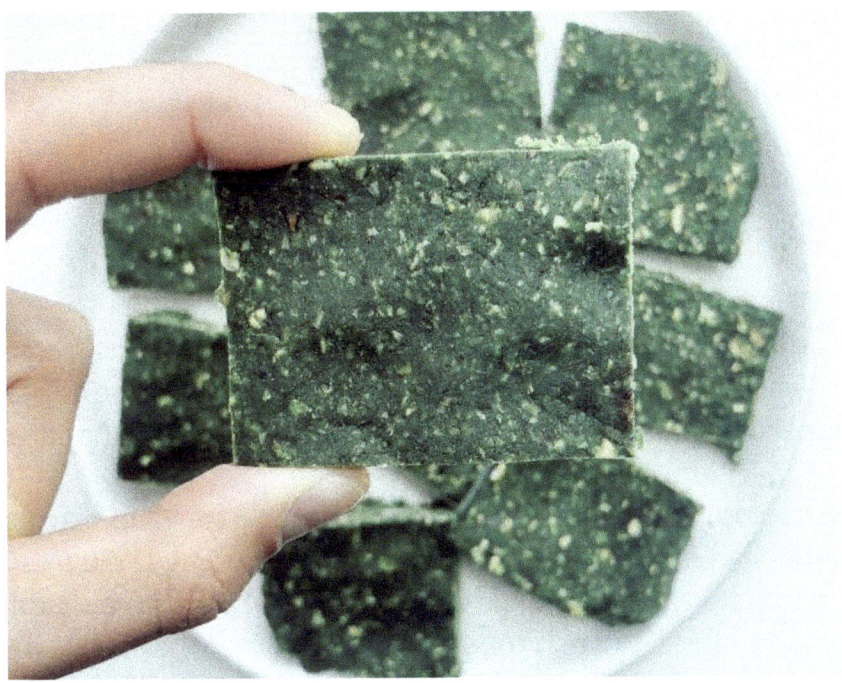

Makes: 8 bars

INGREDIENTS:
- 1 cup Almond Pulp or Almond Flour
- 1 cup Rolled Oats
- 6 Dates remove pits
- 1 teaspoon Spirulina
- 2 ½ tablespoons Coconut Oil

INSTRUCTIONS:
a) Place the oats and coconut oil in a microwave-safe container.
b) Microwave for 1-2 minutes or until the coconut oil melts. It is important to include the oats so that they will slightly heat and get a little crispy. Set aside to cool.
c) Once cooled, remove the pits from the fresh dates and place all ingredients in a food processor. I recommend soaking the dates in advance to help them blend easier. Blend until the mixture is fully blended and starts to stick together. You will need to scoop the mixture off the sides of the food processor several times throughout the blending process.
d) Line a small square dish with parchment paper. Place the mixture on top of the parchment paper and flatten it out until it evenly spreads across the dish. The mixture should be thick and stick together.
e) Place the dish in the fridge to cool for about 30 minutes. Remove from the refrigerator and cut into square bars. Enjoy!

21. Spirulina Protein Bites

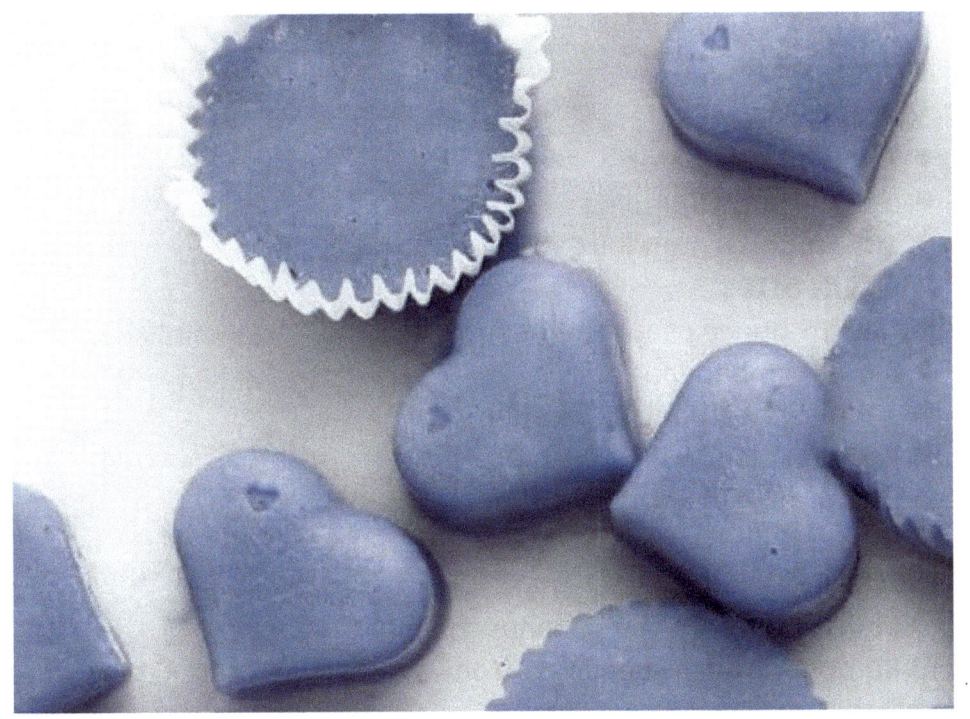

Makes: 6

INGREDIENTS:
BREWED TEA
- 1 cup boiling water
- 1 tablespoon Spirulina
- 1 teaspoon lemon juice

PROTEIN BITES
- Half 15-ounce can white beans
- 3 medium bananas
- 3 tablespoon baobab powder
- ¼-½ cup plant milk
- ½ cup brewed Spirulina tea

INSTRUCTIONS:
a) Chop and freeze the bananas the night before.
b) Remove frozen bananas from freezer at least 20 minutes before.
c) Line a mini-cupcake pan with paper liners.
d) Line up your heart molds on the counter if you are using those.

MAKE BITES
e) Brew the Spirulina tea by adding it to 1 cup of just-boiled hot water for 3 minutes.
f) To a high speed blender, add ½ cup cooled tea, the baobab and the thawed bananas.
g) Open the can of beans, drain and rinse them. Add them to the blender.
h) Lastly add ¼ cup of the milk, and begin blending. Add only enough milk to be sure the texture is creamy but pourable.
i) Add a bit more plant milk if the mixture is not pourable enough to get it into small molds - it all depends on how big your bananas were, and how thick your choice of plant milk is.
j) Taste-test as this point and be sure the mixture is sweet enough for you. If not, you can add a tablespoon or two of maple syrup or

maybe some ripe green grapes. The color will change, but the taste will be sweeter.

k) Pour the mixture into the mini cupcake pan or the silicon heart molds or any vessel you choose to freeze them in.

l) Freeze them at least four hours or until hard enough to remove from the molds; keep them frozen in a freezer-friendly, air-tight container. We've had them at least a month frozen and they still taste wonderful.

22. Spirulina Summer Rolls

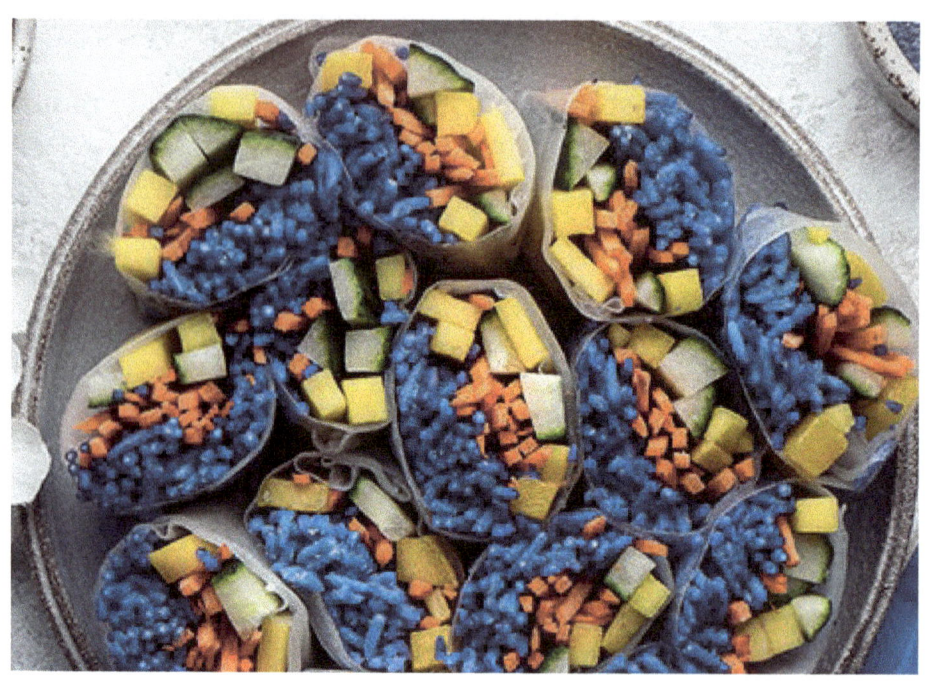

INGREDIENTS:
- 8 oz Rice Noodles:
- 1 tablespoon Blue Spirulina powder
- 2 carrots, sliced thinly
- 2 mini cucumbers, sliced thinly
- Purple cabbage, sliced thinly
- Fresh mint
- Rice paper wrappers

PEANUT SAUCE:
- ¼ cup peanut butter
- 2 tablespoons tamari or soy sauce
- 2 tablespoons water
- 1 tablespoon rice vinegar
- 1 teaspoon coconut sugar
- ½ teaspoon ground ginger
- ½ teaspoon red pepper flakes

INSTRUCTIONS:
a) Bring 8 cups of water to a boil in a large pot. Whisk in Blue Spirulina powder, then add rice noodles.
b) Turn off heat and let noodles steep for 8-10 minutes, until al dente. Drain and rinse with cold water.
c) Whisk together all ingredients for peanut sauce until smooth.
d) Prep all ingredients for summer rolls. Moisten a rice paper wrapper in water for a few seconds, then transfer to a flat surface.
e) Arrange rice noodles and sliced veggies in the bottom center of wrap, leaving space on the right, left and bottom.
f) Fold the right and left sides over the filling, then tuck and roll from the bottom up to enclose the filling.
g) Repeat with remaining rice paper wrappers and filling.
h) Slice in half and enjoy with peanut sauce!

23. Spirulina Cupcakes

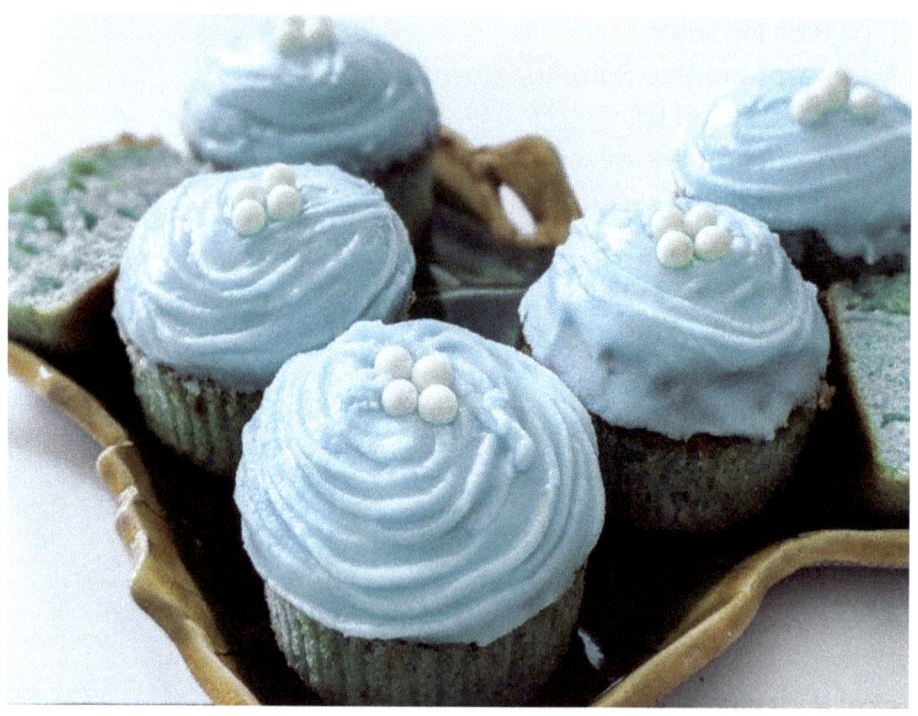

Makes: 12 servings

INGREDIENTS:
- 1 ¾ cup all-purpose flour
- ¾ teaspoon salt
- ½ teaspoon baking soda
- 1 ½ teaspoon baking powder
- ½ cup vegetable oil
- 1 cup sugar
- 2 eggs, beaten
- ⅓ cup sourdough surplus, about
- ½ cup buttermilk
- 1-2 tablespoons Spirulina powder
- 2 teaspoon vanilla extract
- 2 teaspoon lemon juice, fresh

BUTTERCREAM ICING
- 227 g room temperature butter, about 1 cup
- 400 g icing sugar, about 2 cups
- 5 g vanilla, 1 teaspoon
- 28 g cream 18%, about 2-4 tablespoons

INSTRUCTIONS:
a) Preheat oven to 350 degrees Fahrenheit and line cupcake pan with cupcake liners. If not using liners spray pan with oil.
b) In one bowl combine flour, baking powder, baking soda, and salt. Set aside.
c) Crack room temp eggs in separate small bowl set aside.
d) In a large bowl with whisk, or in standard mixer with whisk attachment combine sugar, oil, buttermilk, sourdough surplus, mix for 1 minute until well combined. Add eggs and vanilla continue to mix for an additional minute.
e) Pour in pea flower, mix until batter is smooth and even color.
f) Add flour mixture and continue to blend for about a minute.

g) For the last step you will be mixing with a spoon to insure you are not over beating the batter.

h) Add lemon juice and stir well with spoon. You should notice the color of the batter changing from a green/blue, to deeper richer blue. Blend with spoon until color is even and lemon juice is dispersed.

i) Pour batter into cupcake pan and bake at 350 for 18-20 minutes.

j) Buttercream Icing

k) With standard, or hand held mixer, using whisk or paddle attachment whip room temperature salted butter on medium high for 2-3 minutes, or until it is smooth and creamy.

l) Add the icing sugar.

m) Once sugar is incorporated mix on high for 3-4 minutes, adding vanilla, followed by the cream. Start with 2 tablespoons of cream, if you want a thinner icing then just add more cream. For decorating these cupcakes, I like to use between 2-3 tablespoons cream.

n) Continue to whip for another 2-4 minutes, until your buttercream is light and fluffy.

o) Scoop buttercream into piping bag and decorate, fully cooled, cupcakes.

p) Bake on through to the other side

24. Spirulina Glazed donuts

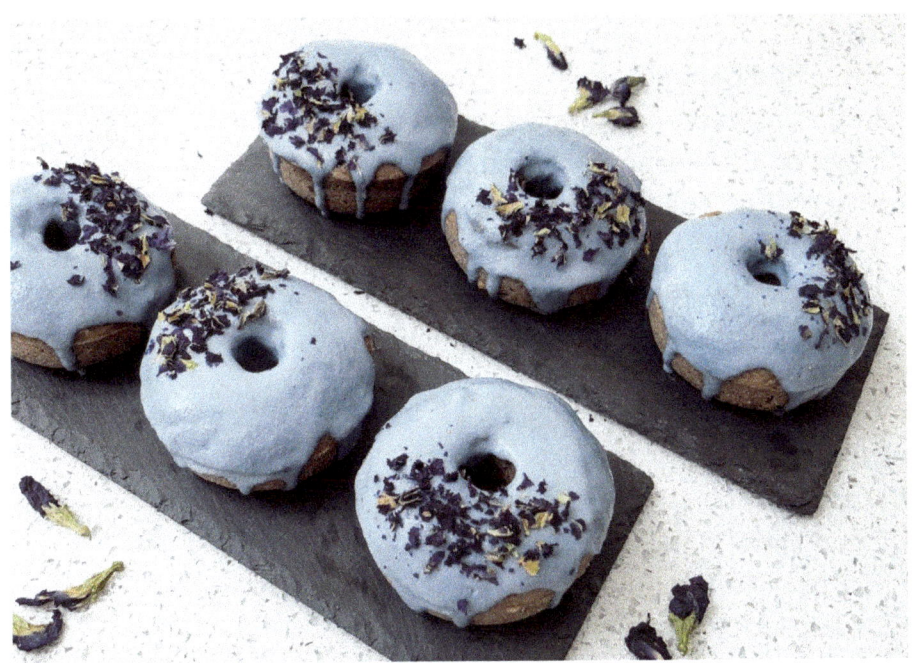

INGREDIENTS:
DONUT:
- 1 mashed banana
- 1 cup unsweetened apple sauce
- 1 egg or 1 tablespoon chia seeds mixed with water
- 50 g melted coconut oil
- 4 tablespoons honey or agave nectar syrup
- 1 tablespoon vanilla
- 1 teaspoon cinnamon
- 150 g buckwheat flour
- 1 teaspoon baking powder

Spirulina GLAZE:
- ½ cup cashews, soaked 4 hours
- 1 cup almond milk
- 40 Spirulina tea flowers
- 1 tablespoon agave nectar syrup
- 1 tablespoon vanilla essence

INSTRUCTIONS:
TO MAKE THE DONUTS:
a) Mix all the dry ingredients together.
b) Mix all the wet ingredients together.
c) Add the wet to the dry and then transfer to the donut molds.
d) Bake at 160 degrees for 15 minutes.

TO MAKE THE GLAZE:
e) Blend the cashews in a food processor until smooth.
f) In a saucepan, heat the almond milk and add the tea. Simmer on a low heat for 10 minutes.
g) Add the blue almond milk to the blended cashews, add the agave nectar and vanilla essence and blend again until combined.
h) Keep refrigerated until your donuts have cooked & cooled.
i) Decorate the donuts with the glaze and extra flowers!
j) These donuts are vegan and gluten & refined sugar free – so really there's no need to hold back: go ahead and eat them all!

25. Spirulina Peanut Mochi

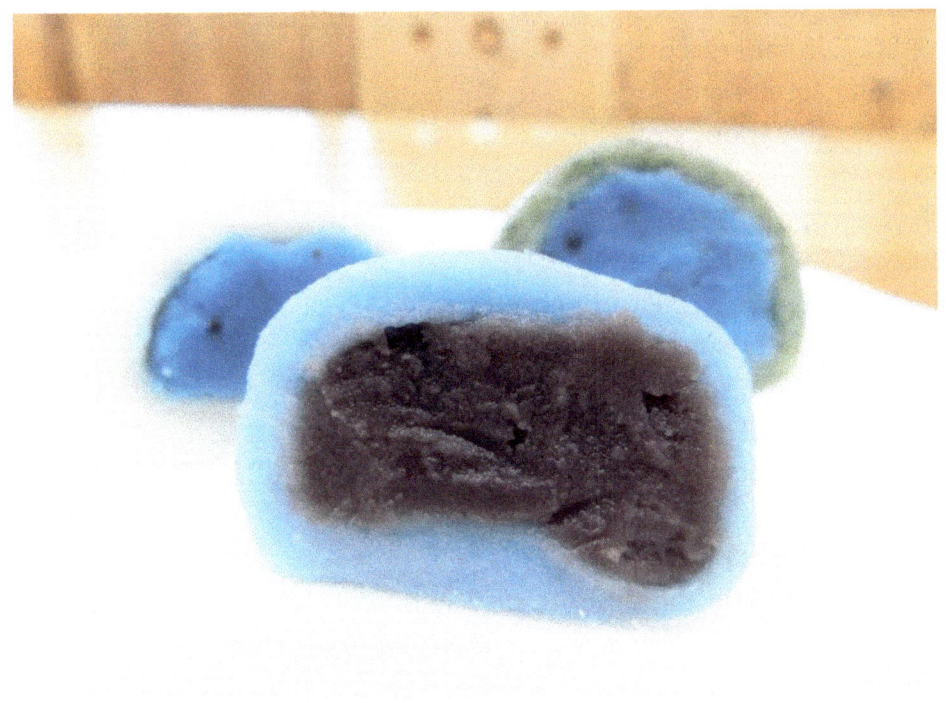

INGREDIENTS:
MOCHI:
- 300g glutinous rice flour
- 50g wheat starch
- 75g caster sugar
- 1 ½ tablespoons oil
- 450ml water
- ½ teaspoon Spirulina powder

PEANUT FILLING:
- 300g blended roasted peanuts
- 100g caster sugar
- ¼ teaspoon salt

FLOUR FOR COATING & DUSTING:
- 200g rice flour, fried for 20 min over medium heat.

INSTRUCTIONS:
a) Mix all mochi ingredients until well combined. Sieve and pour into a greased steaming tray and steam over medium heat for 25 min.

b) When the rice flour mixture is cool enough to handle, scrape it out onto a work surface scattered lightly with the dusting flour.

c) Divide cooking dough into small portion, about 35-40g each using sharp knife dusted in flour.

d) Working with one piece at a time and dusting your hands with flour to stop it sticking, roll each piece into a ball.

e) Flatten the ball then use your hands to form it into a round 8 cm across.

f) Mix all filling ingredients, then place a tablespoon of the filling in the centre of the round then bring the edges over the filling to enclose, pinching them together well to seal.

g) Gently re-roll into a round, pressing the top slightly to flatten a little.

h) Coated the Mochi with flour to smoothen the surface.

i) Mochi will keep stored in an airtight container for up to 2 days.

26. Blueberry Spirulina Muffins

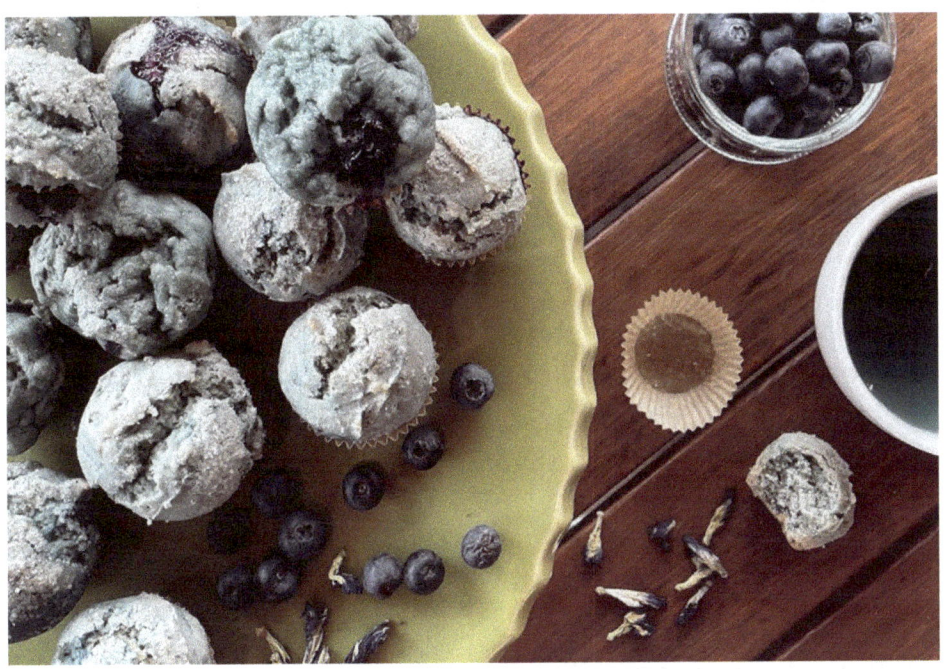

INGREDIENTS
WET:
- ½ cup Spirulina
- 1 teaspoon lemon zest
- ½ cup whole milk, warm
- 1 stick unsalted butter, melted
- 2 eggs

DRY:
- 2-½ cup all-purpose gluten-free flour
- 2 teaspoons baking powder
- ¼ teaspoon baking soda
- 1 cup white granulated sugar
- 1 teaspoon Kosher Salt
- 1 cup fresh blueberries

INSTRUCTIONS:
a) Preheat your oven to 350 degrees.
b) In a blender. add all of the wet ingredients and let them sit for ten minutes, then blend until smooth.
c) The mixture will turn indigo from the Spirulina and look slightly thick from the melted butter. Set it aside.
d) In a large bowl add the gluten-free flour, baking powder, baking soda, sugar and kosher salt and give it a mix.
e) Reserve a quarter cup of the dry mixture and toss the blueberries until coated, set them aside. This will absorb any excess moisture and prevent them from altering the batter's consistency.
f) Meanwhile, in a large bowl, stir the wet ingredients into the dry ingredients using a spatula. The mixture will vary in blue hues and that's okay. Once the batter looks combined, sprinkle in the blueberries, then fold them in gently.
g) Assemble your mini muffins tins with muffin liners.
h) Using a scoop, fill the mini muffin tins ¾ of the way full.

i) Bake muffins for 10 minutes or until an inserted toothpick comes out clean.

27. Spirulina Granola Bars

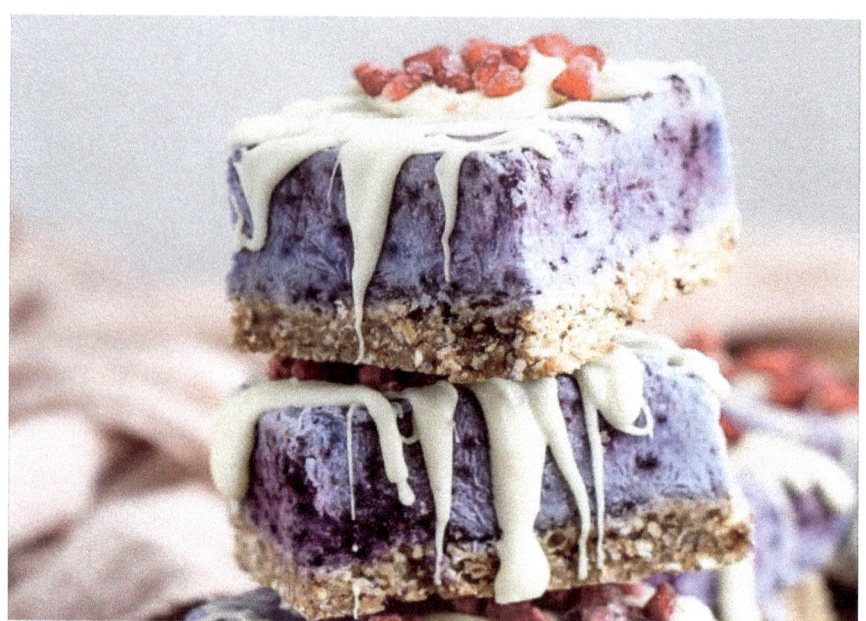

Makes: 4 servings

INGREDIENTS:
- 2 cups rolled oats, gluten-free if desired
- 1 cup Pepitas
- 1 ½ cups unsweetened puffed rice cereal
- ½ cup dried fruit, roughly chopped
- ¼ teaspoons flaky sea salt
- 1½ tablespoons Spirulina powder
- ⅓ cup brown rice syrup
- 3 tablespoons maple syrup
- ½ cup tahini
- 2 tablespoons coconut oil
- 1 teaspoon vanilla extract

INSTRUCTIONS:
a) Preheat oven to 325°F/160°C.
b) Combine oats and pepitas on a baking sheet and bake for 10-15 minutes, stirring once or twice, until the oats are golden and have a nutty aroma.
c) In a small saucepan combine the brown rice syrup, maple syrup, tahini, coconut oil, and vanilla.
d) Whisk to combine. Do not overheat.
e) In a large bowl, combine the cooled oats and pumpkin seeds with the chopped dried fruit, rice puffs, salt, and Spirulina powder.
f) Pour the wet ingredients over the dry ingredients and stir quickly to mix.
g) Pour the mix into a brownie pan lined with plastic wrap or baking paper. Press the mixture firmly, especially into the corners.
h) Place in the fridge for a couple of hours to firm up, then remove from fridge and slice into bars. Keep leftovers in the fridge for up two weeks.

28. Spirulina Lime Popcorn

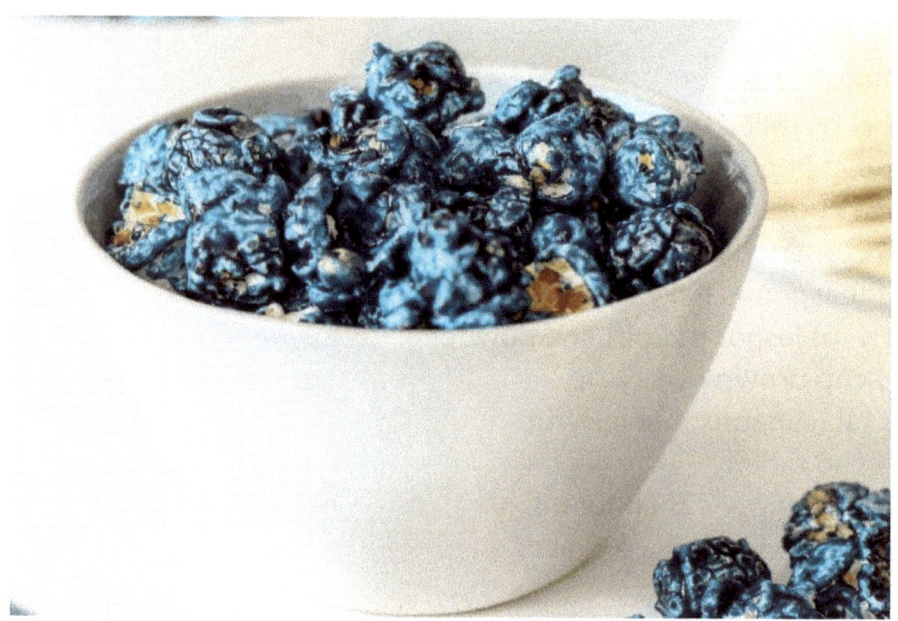

Makes: 2 servings

INGREDIENTS
- 1 tablespoon coconut oil
- ¼ cup popcorn kernels
- 2 tablespoon sugar
- 1 tablespoon vegan butter
- ½ teaspoon water
- 1 teaspoon Spirulina powder
- 1 teaspoon very finely chopped lime zest

INSTRUCTIONS

a) Heat the oil in a large and deep pot or saucepan over medium heat.

b) Add a couple of popcorn kernels to the pot and wait for them to pop.

c) Once they have popped, add the rest of the popcorn kernels, stir to coat with oil, and remove from heat. Wait 30-50 seconds and put the pot back on the stove.

d) Cover with a lid and wait for the kernels to pop. Once it starts to pop, shake the pot a few times to make sure all the kernels cook evenly. Continue cooking until all the kernels have popped. Remove from heat and transfer to a large mixing bowl.

e) Add the sugar and vegan butter to a small saucepan. Feel free to add a pinch of salt as well. Heat over medium heat and let it boil for about 1 minute. Add the water, stir, and cook for another 20 seconds, or until the sugar is fully dissolved.

f) Pour over the popcorn while stirring at the same time to coat it evenly with the syrup.

g) Sift the Spirulina over the popcorn and stir to coat. Add the lime zests and stir again.

h) Serve immediately.

29. Spirulina Almond Crescents

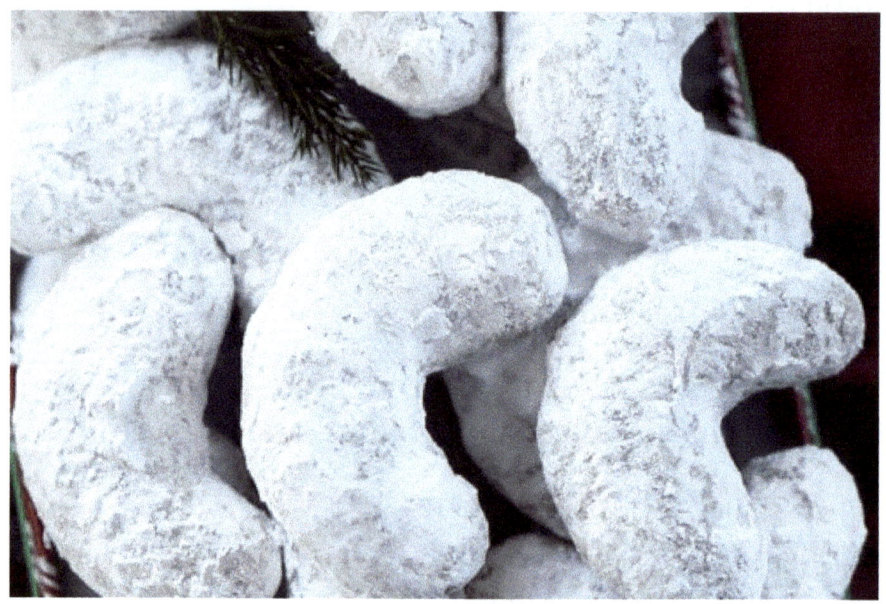

Makes: 3 Dozen Cookies

INGREDIENTS
SPIRULINA DOUGH:
- ½ Cup Vegan Butter
- ½ Cup Smooth Almond Butter
- ⅔ Cup Granulated Sugar
- 3 Tablespoons Vegan Vanilla Yogurt
- 1 Tablespoon Spirulina Powder
- 1 Teaspoon Vanilla Extract
- ½ Teaspoon Almond Extract
- 2 Cups All-Purpose Flour
- 1 Cup Blanched Almond Flour
- ¼ Teaspoon Salt

TO FINISH:
- ½ Confectioner's Sugar

INSTRUCTIONS
a) Using your stand mixer with the paddle attachment installed, cream together the butter, almond butter, sugar, yogurt, spirulina, vanilla, and almond extract.
b) Mix until completely homogeneous, light, and fluffy.
c) In a separate bowl, whisk together both flours and salt. Gradually add the dry ingredients with the motor on the lowest possible speed, until fully incorporated. Pause to scrape down the sides of the bowl as needed.
d) Scoop out about small balls of dough for each cookie, and roll between lightly moistened hands to shape into cylinders. Press with gentle force on the outer ends to turn them into more pointed horns, and bend into crescent shapes.
e) Place approximately 1 inch apart on ungreased baking sheets, and bake for 22 - 26 minutes, or until set and bottoms are lightly browned. Let stand for 2 - 3 minutes before removing to wire racks to cool completely.

f) Toss with confectioner's sugar to coat. Serve or stash in the freezer for up to 3 months.

MAIN COURSE

30. Mermaid Pasta

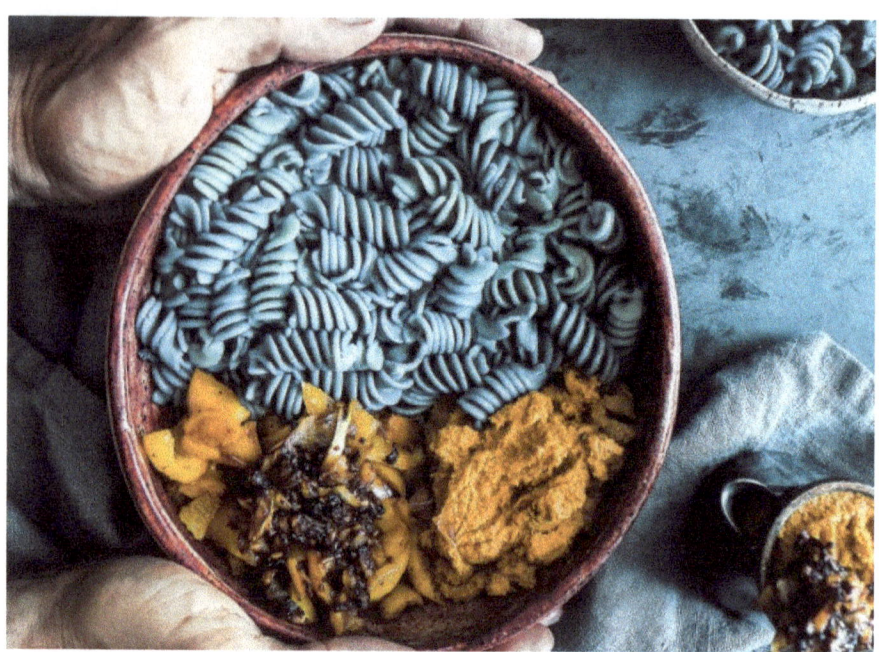

Makes: 2 servings

INGREDIENTS:
- 1 cup canned pumpkin
- 2 cups Pasta of your choice
- ½ cup veggie stock
- ½ cup coconut milk
- 2 Tablespoons tahini
- Juice of 1 lemon
- ½ onion caramelized
- 1 bell pepper
- 1 tablespoon garlic
- 1 teaspoon pumpkin pie spice
- 1 teaspoon onion powder
- 1 teaspoon coconut sugar
- Salt & pepper
- 1 teaspoon blue spirulina

INSTRUCTIONS:
a) Caramelize your onion in some coconut oil. Add in garlic halfway through and 1 teaspoon of coconut sugar.
b) Add water to your pan with 1 teaspoon of blue spirulina to the water before bringing it to a boil
c) Cook your pasta according to the packet.
d) Add pumpkin, coconut milk, lemon juice, tahini, and spices to a pan and cook for 5 minutes on low heat.
e) Assemble everything however you like afterward and snap a pic!
f) If your pasta doesn't take the color, remove it from heat add more spirulina, and let it soak for a few minutes and that usually does the trick

31. Corn Fish Tacos with Spirulina Blue Rice & Crema

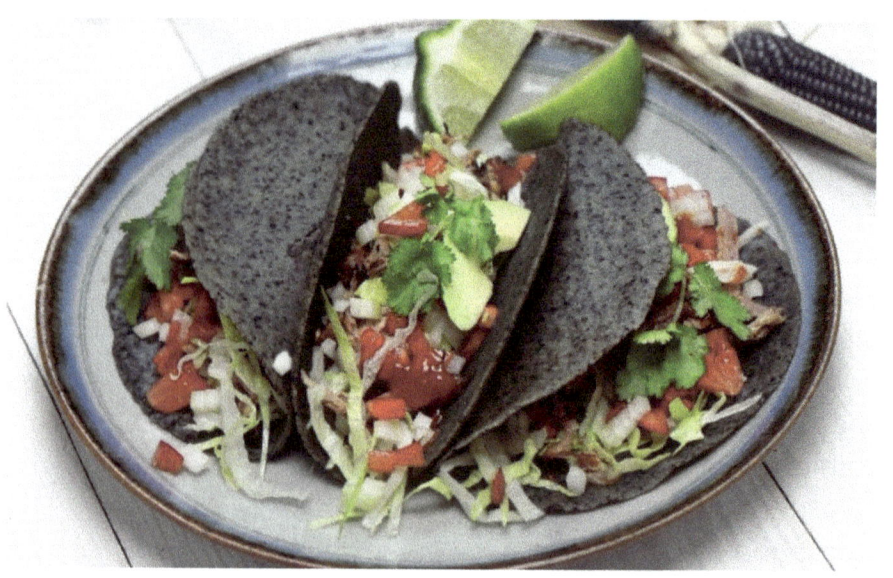

Makes: 8 tacos

INGREDIENTS:
FOR THE FISH
- 1½ pounds flaky white fish, skinned, boned, and cleaned
- ¼ teaspoon salt
- ¼ teaspoon pepper
- 1 teaspoon ground cumin
- Avocado oil or other neutral cooking oil
- Zest of 1 lime

FOR THE BLUE RICE
- 2 cups cooked white rice
- ½ gram blue spirulina powder
- 1 tablespoon finely chopped fresh cilantro
- 1 tablespoon fresh lime juice
- Neutral oil, like avocado oil
- ⅛ teaspoon salt
- Pinch of black pepper

FOR THE BLUE CREMA
- ¾ cup Mexican crema, sour cream, or Greek yogurt
- ½ cup mayonnaise
- ½ gram blue spirulina powder
- 1 large clove of garlic, grated on a Microplane or minced
- 2 tablespoons fresh lime juice
- ⅛ teaspoon salt

TO SERVE
- Corn Tacos

INSTRUCTIONS
MAKE THE FISH:
a) Preheat oven to 375°.
b) Season fish on both sides with salt, black pepper, and cumin.
c) Drizzle with a neutral oil, and bake until cooked through or until internal temperature reaches 145°. Remove from oven, and

sprinkle lime zest evenly on top. Break up fish into large chunks for tacos, and set them aside for assembly.

d) Mix cooked rice with blue spirulina, cilantro, lime juice, a drizzle of neutral oil, and salt and pepper. Toss until evenly mixed, taste for seasoning, and set aside for taco assembly.

e) Mix all crema ingredients in a small bowl, and chill in the refrigerator for taco assembly.

f) Place a small scoop of blue rice on each blue corn tortilla. Top with a little shredded cabbage, some fish pieces, a dollop of blue crema, and a sprinkle of crushed blue corn tortilla chips.

32. **Blue Risotto with White Fish**

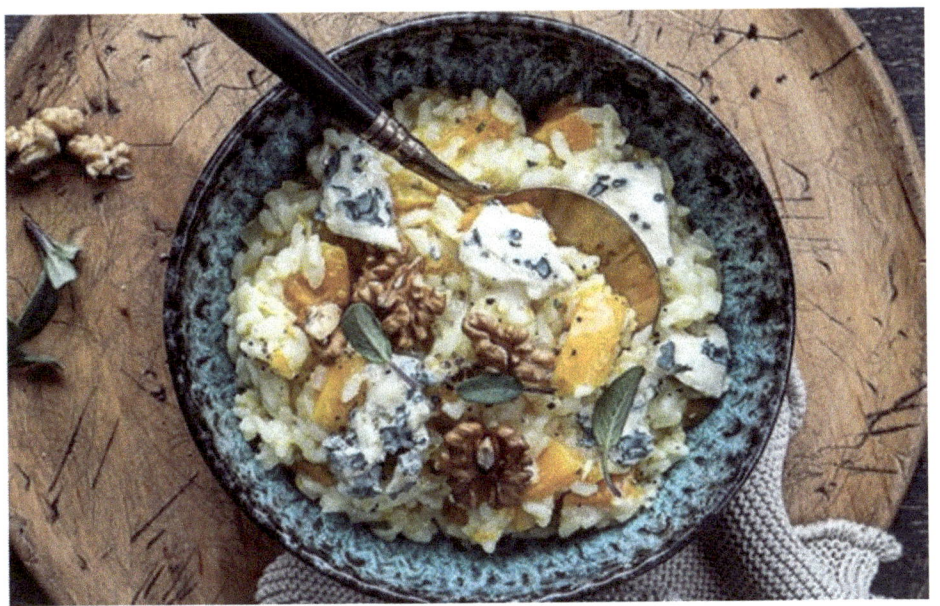

Makes: 2 Servings

INGREDIENTS:
- 180g Acquerello rice
- 150g of Branzino
- 1 Tablespoon of Dried Scallops
- 3 Teaspoons of Organic Blue Spirulina Powder
- 1 Spring Onion
- Extra-virgin Olive Oil
- Black Pepper
- Sea Salt
- Organic Kitchen

INSTRUCTIONS
a) Soak the dried scallops in freshly boiled water for 25-30mins. Pour the water and the dried scallops into a small saucepan and pre-heat it.
b) Slice the spring onion and simmer it with extra-virgin olive oil in a pot. Once the oil is warm and the spring onion starts to sizzle, add the rice and toast it for a couple of minutes.
c) Start pouring small amounts of the water with the dried scallops into the pot with the rice and continue stirring. Keep doing this for three-quarters of the rice cooking time.
d) Season with sea salt and black pepper. Add the branzino and continue stirring for a couple of minutes, adding water to prevent the rice from sticking to the pot.
e) Make sure you add the right amount of water to make the risotto creamy.
f) Add 3 teaspoons of blue spirulina powder in a glass with 100g of water and whisk until the powder is fully mixed and smooth. Add the blue water to the risotto and mix it all.
g) Once the risotto is finally cooked, add sea salt and freshly ground to taste and drizzle some extra-virgin olive oil.

33. Sea Brim with Rice and Spirulina

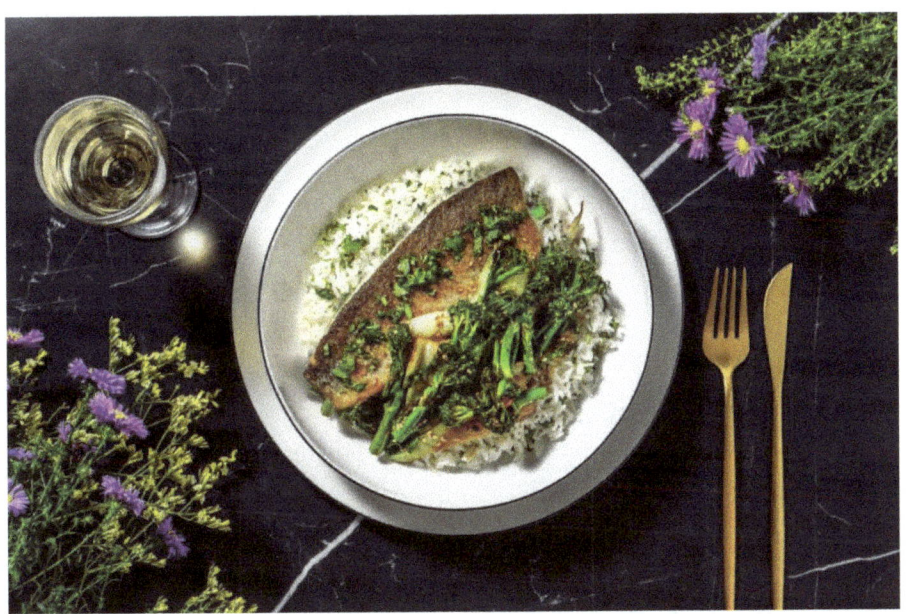

Makes: 2

INGREDIENTS
- 4 Sea Brims
- 2 cups Rice
- ½ teaspoon Spirulina
- Salt
- Pepper
- Olive Oil
- Dill, to garnish
- Pomegranate, to garnish

INSTRUCTIONS
a) Put the rice to boil in a pot with plenty of salted water.
b) After about 10 minutes, strain it, and it's ready.
c) As the rice is boiling, warm up an anti-stick pan and drizzle some olive oil on it.
d) Grill the fish fillets, placing the skin on the bottom first.
e) Grill for 4-5 minutes and turn it on the other side.
f) After 2 minutes switch the fire off and leave the fish on the stove for another 5 minutes.
g) Remove it from the fire and leave it on the side.
h) Once the rice is ready and still hot sprinkle some spirulina powder on top and mix it lightly using a fork so that it goes everywhere and all of your rice is now colored.
i) Serve after garnishing with some fresh dill and some pomegranate.

34. Spirulina Vegetable Fried Rice

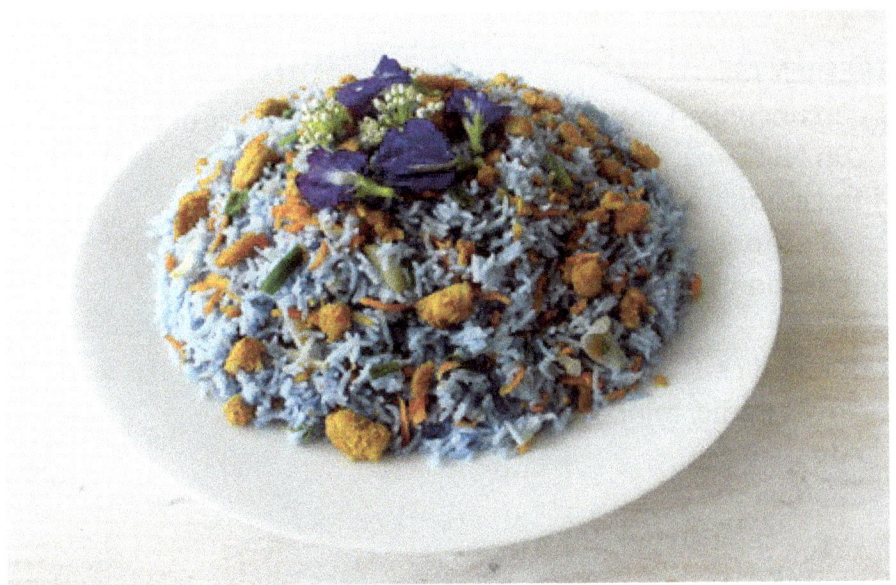

Makes: 2-3 Servings

INGREDIENTS:
- 1 cup uncooked short grain rice, makes 3 cups cooked
- 1 cup water
- ¼ teaspoon Blue Spirulina powder
- 2 tablespoons oil
- ¾ teaspoon salt and Pepper

VEGGIES:
- 1 onion, diced
- 2 cloves garlic, minced
- ½ cup corn
- ½ cup peas
- ½ cup diced carrots

CHOPPED KALE
- 1 red bell pepper, diced
- 1 cup chopped purple cabbage

INSTRUCTIONS:
a) Wash the rice through running water 2 to 3 times. In a rice cooker, add in the water, washed rice, and Blue Spirulina powder.
b) Leave to cook and then cool for 15 minutes. Cooling the rice prevents it from being too sticky and mushy when stir-frying!
c) In a large pan or skillet, heat 2 tablespoons oil. Add in the chopped onion and garlic. Sauté until cooked through and garlic is lightly brown. Add in the rest of the veggies. Season with ¾ teaspoon salt, or to taste and some pepper. Mix in the cooled rice.
d) Leave to cook for 3 to 4 minutes over medium high heat.
e) Serve and enjoy!

35. Spirulina Dumplings

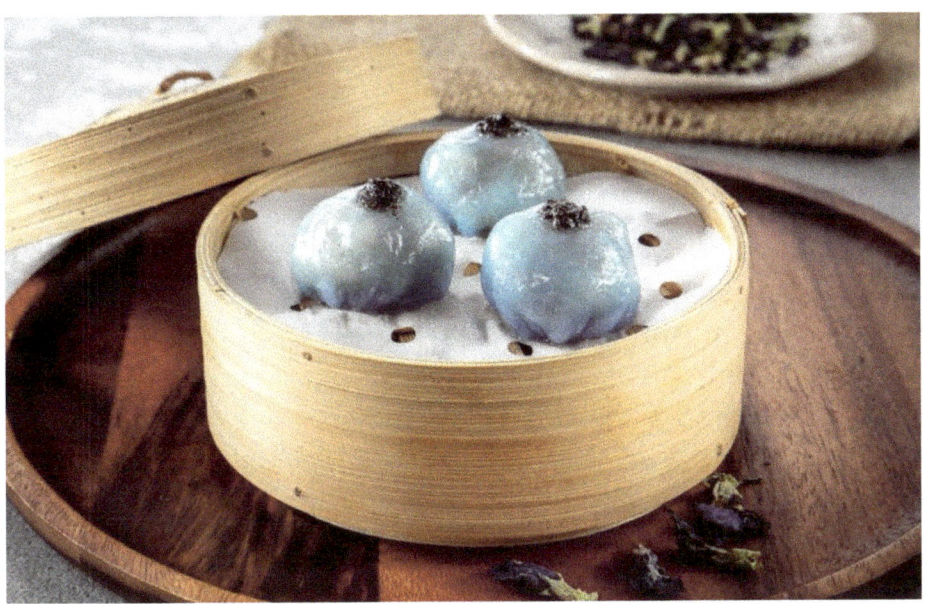

INGREDIENTS:
WRAPPERS:
- 2 cups all-purpose flour
- 1 cup boiling water
- ½ teaspoon Blue Spirulina powder, dissolved in 1 teaspoon water
- 1 teaspoon Rose Salt

FILLING:
- 100g enoki mushroom
- 70g shredded carrot
- 25g rehydrated & shredded black fungus
- 100g cabbage
- ½ tablespoons freshly greater ginger
- 2 teaspoon minced garlic
- 2 teaspoon cornstarch
- ½ teaspoon ground pepper
- 1 tablespoon toasted sesame oil
- ¼ teaspoon Rose Salt

INSTRUCTIONS:
a) In a stand mixer, add flour, salt and water, knead until you have a smooth dough. Remove half of the dough from the mixer, set aside. Add Spirulina powder into the half dough and continue kneading until combined. Let doughs rest for 20 minutes.

b) Bring 2 cup water to boil, add enoki mushrooms and cook for 2 minutes. Sprinkle 2 pinches of salt onto the cabbage and mix well with your hands. Allow this to sit for minutes. Squeeze out excess water. Add sesame oil into a pan and heat over medium heat until hot. Add the garlic and ginger. Stir a few times to release the fragrance. Add the carrot, black fungus, stir and cook for 1 minute.

c) Add the cabbage & enoki mushrooms cook and stir for another 1 minute. Add in salt, pepper and dissolved cornstarch, stir until all the liquid has evaporated. Transfer to a big plate to cool.

d) Fill and seal the dumplings. Heat the oil in a large frying pan over medium heat. Fry the dumplings flat side down for about 2 minutes until a golden crust forms on the bottom. Add the ¼ cup water and immediately cover with a lid and let the steam cook the dumplings for 8 minutes or until all the water has evaporated.
e) Remove the lid and let the dumplings to cook for a further minute until they lift off from the bottom of the pan easily.

SALAD

36. Spirulina Sea Salad

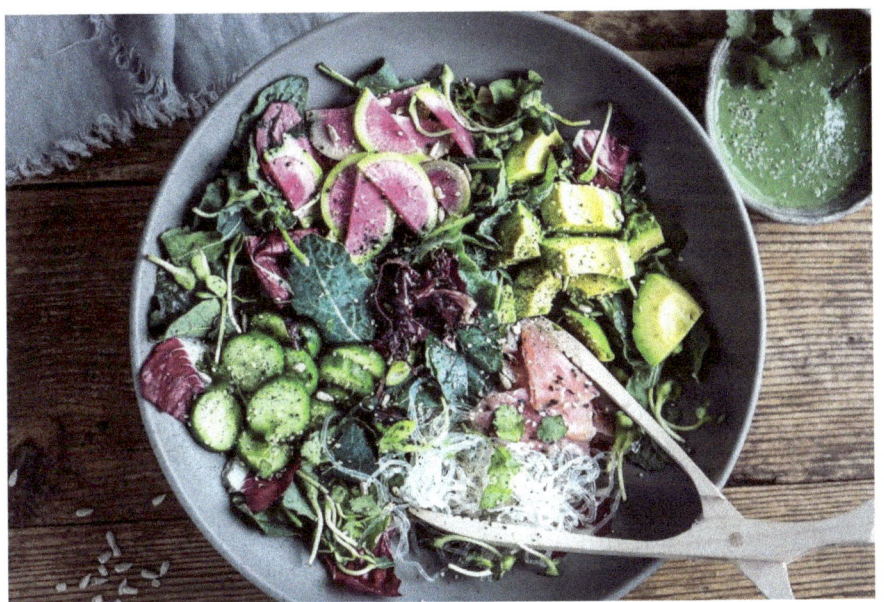

Makes: 3-4

INGREDIENTS:
- ¼ cup dulse ribbons, soaked in water
- 4 ounces of baby kale
- 1 Turkish cucumber, sliced
- 1 avocado, diced or sliced
- 1–2 green onions
- 1 cup Kelp noodles
- 1–2 watermelon radishes, thinly sliced
- Smoked ahi, smoked salmon, baked or smoked tofu, edamame

GARNISH:
- Sunflower Sprouts
- Hemp seeds or sunflower seeds
- Cilantro or edible flower petals

SPIRULINA DRESSING:
- ¼ cup water
- ⅓ cup olive oil
- ¼ cup hemp seeds
- 3 tablespoons Apple Cider vinegar
- 1 garlic clove
- ¾ teaspoon salt
- ¼ teaspoon cracked pepper
- ½ cup cilantro
- 1 teaspoon spirulina, more to taste

INSTRUCTIONS

a) Soak the dulse ribbons in a small bowl of water, for 15 minutes or until softened

b) Make the Spirulina dressing– add all but the cilantro and spirulina to a blender, and blend until creamy and smooth- a full minute. Add cilantro and spirulina, and pulse until well combined and smooth.

c) Add the salad ingredients to a bowl- greens first then cucumber, avocado, scallions, kelp noodles, radishes, drained dulse, and your choice of protein.
d) Toss with some of the dressing, just enough to coat.
e) Garnish with seeds and sprouts.

37. Spirulina Zucchini Noodle Salad

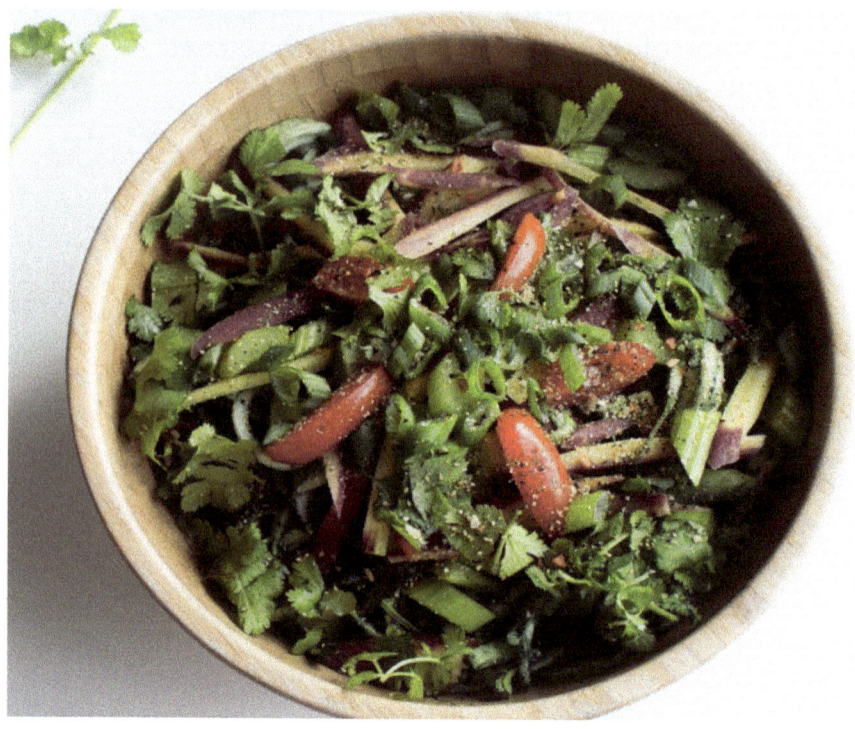

Makes: 1 salad

INGREDIENTS:
- 1 small-medium zucchini
- 2 celery sticks, chopped
- 1 carrot, chopped
- 6 grape tomatoes, quartered
- 1 green onion, chopped
- 1 teaspoon spirulina
- juice from ½ a lemon
- 1 teaspoon extra virgin olive oil or ¼ of an avocado
- garlic powder and/or Mrs. Dash to taste
- 1 tablespoon nutritional yeast
- pinch of salt

INSTRUCTIONS
a) Spiralize or peel zucchini into ribbons. Toss with seasonings, spirulina, nutritional yeast, extra virgin olive oil, lemon juice, and salt.
b) Top with remaining veggies.

38. Kale, Apple & Pecan Salad with Spirulina dressing

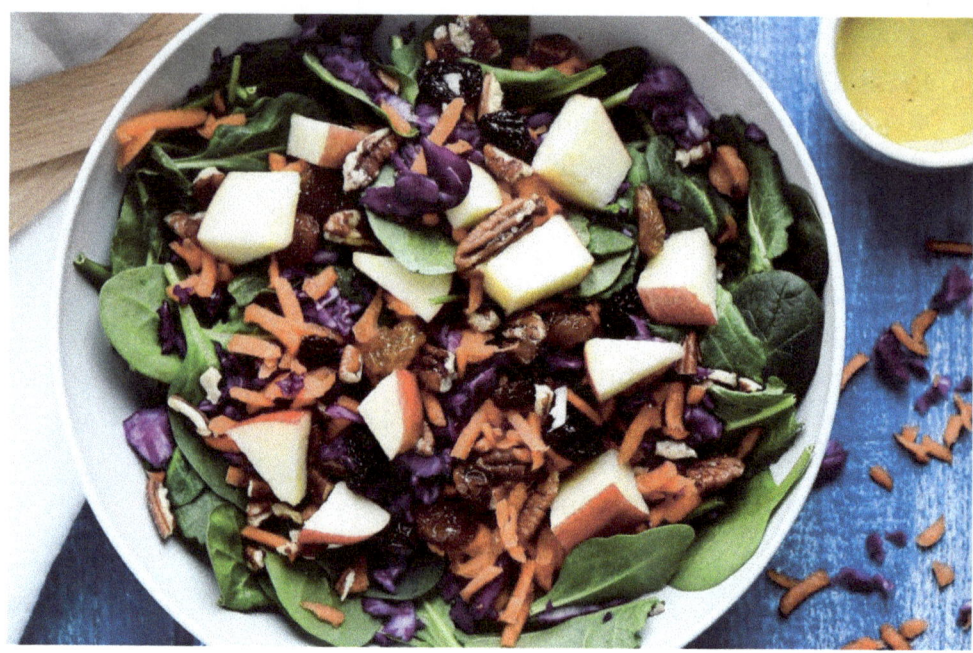

Makes: 4 servings

INGREDIENTS:
SALAD
- 1 small box of mixed organic Greens
- 1 bunch Kale
- 1 – 2 pieces Apples - cut up into bite chunks
- ½ cup roasted or dehydrated Pecans

SPIRULINA HEMP DRESSING
- ¼ cup cold pressed Olive Oil
- ½ juice of Lemon
- ¼ cup Hemp Seeds
- 1 teaspoon Spirulina
- 1 tablespoon raw Apple Cider Vinegar
- 3 tablespoons Agave
- 1 clove Garlic
- pinch Himalayan Sea Salt

INSTRUCTIONS:
a) Toss all the salad ingredients.
b) Throw all dressing ingredients in a blender until mixed well.
c) Pour onto the salad. Keep rest in the fridge in a glass bottle or air-tight container.

39. Spirulina Spinach Salad

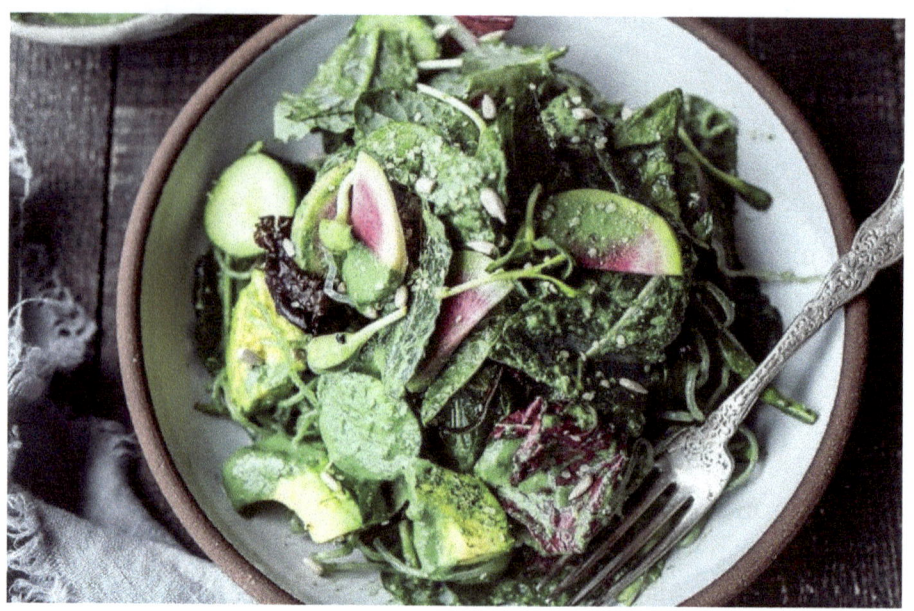

Makes: 4 servings

INGREDIENTS:
- 2 large bowls of baby spinach leaves
- 1 large tomato diced
- 1-2 ripe avocados
- 2 handfuls of sunflower or clover sprouts
- ½ teaspoons of spirulina powder to start
- Splash of olive oil
- Sea salt to taste

INSTRUCTIONS:
a) Add spinach to a bowl and toss in the tomato, avocado, and sprouts.
b) Start with ½ teaspoons of spirulina powder, a splash of olive oil, and a bit of salt.

40. Spirulina Tofu Salad

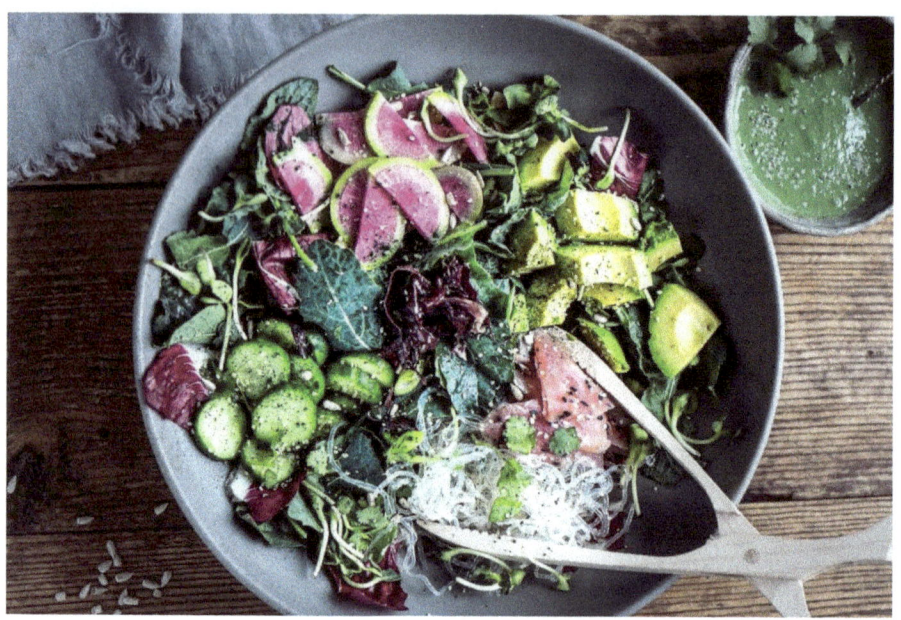

Makes: 4 servings

INGREDIENTS:
- 8 ounces of firm tofu
- 1 bell pepper
- 2 medium tomatoes
- 1 medium zucchini
- 1 medium grated carrot
- 2 stalks celery
- 2 spring onions, finely chopped
- 1 tablespoon tamari or soy sauce
- Generous pinch of basil, thyme, and marjoram
- Hot pepper sauce or cayenne pepper
- 1 heaped teaspoon Spirulina

INSTRUCTIONS:
a) Mix all ingredients together.
b) Almost any combination of raw vegetables can be put into a tofu salad.

SOUPS AND STEW

41. Pea soup with spirulina

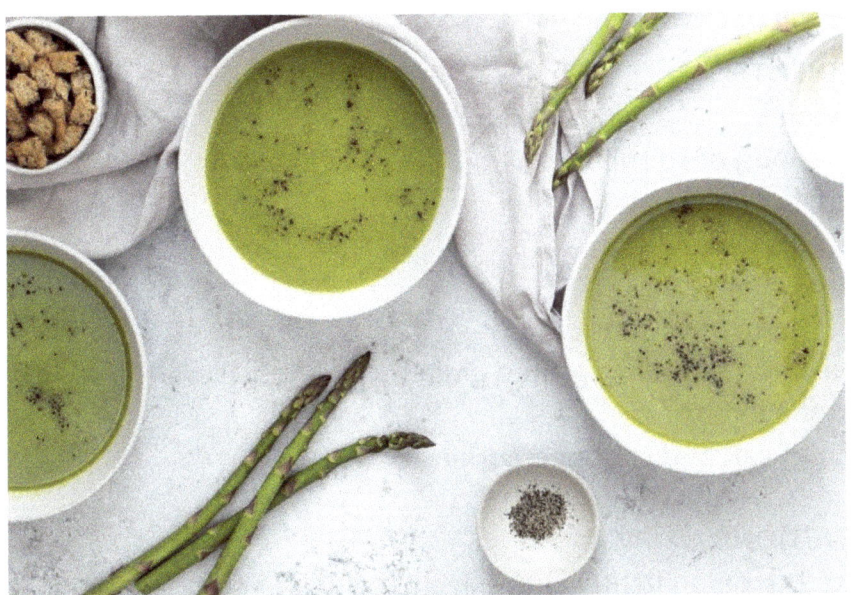

Makes: 2 servings

INGREDIENTS:
- 1 onion
- 1 teaspoon of spirulina
- 1 drizzle of olive oil
- 1 cup of peas
- ½ cup coconut milk
- 1 teaspoon of turmeric
- 1 teaspoon of freshly grated ginger
- Zest of a lemon
- Pinch of salt and chopped coriander

INSTRUCTIONS:
a) Sauté the onion lightly with olive oil, ginger, and turmeric.
b) Add the peas and continue cooking over low heat until the peas are tender.
c) Add the coconut milk and a little bit of water just to cover the peas.
d) Let it cool and blend it finally adding spirulina.
e) Adjust salt and texture with a little bit of water or if you prefer more coconut milk. Serve with chopped coriander and lime zest.

42. Coconut Super greens & Spirulina Soup

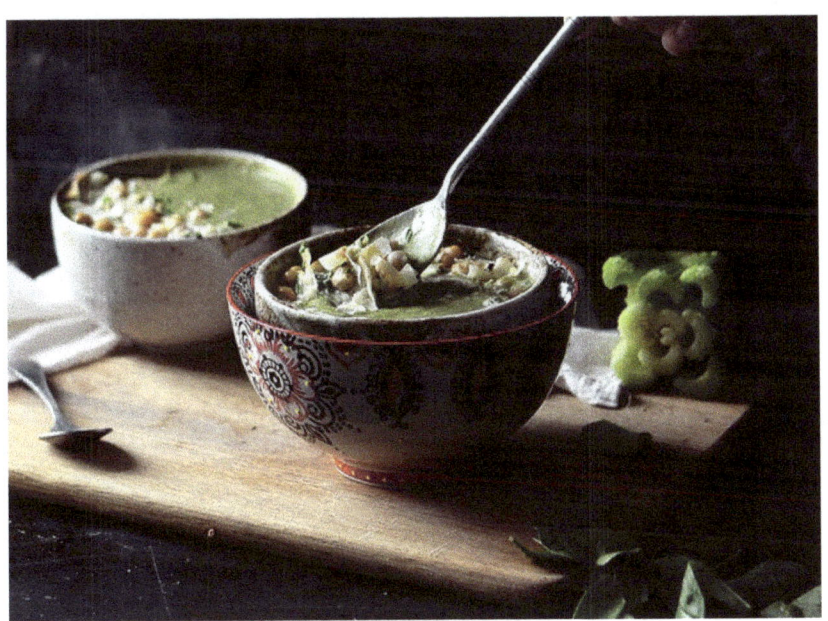

Makes: 5-6

INGREDIENTS:
- 1 teaspoon fennel seeds
- 1 teaspoon caraway seeds
- 2" inches of ginger, chopped
- 3 cloves of garlic, chopped
- 1 large white onion, roughly chopped
- 2 sticks of celery, roughly chopped
- 1 head of broccoli
- 1 courgette/zucchini, chopped
- 1 apple, peeled and chopped
- 2 packed cups of spinach
- 3 cups vegetable stock
- 1 teaspoon sea salt
- 1 teaspoon pepper
- 2 teaspoons spirulina
- 1 tablespoon lime juice

INSTRUCTIONS:
a) Heat 1 tablespoon of olive oil in a large pot over med-high and add the caraway and fennel seeds, and heat until they start popping.
b) Add the onions to the pan and cook for about 3 minutes or until translucent.
c) Add the garlic and ginger and continue to fry for 30 seconds, so it's fragrant.
d) Add the celery and broccoli, stir to combine everything, and cook for 1 minute before adding the apple, courgette, salt, pepper, and vegetable stock.
e) Bring the stock to a boil and then reduce it to a simmer. Simmer for about 10 minutes or until the veggies are tender.
f) Add the coconut milk and bring it back to a simmer.

g) Add the spinach, stir in and cook for 1 minute, until wilted and vibrant green.

h) Remove from the heat and stir in the lime juice and spirulina.

i) Transfer to a blender and whizz on high until smooth! Top with croutons, roasted chickpeas, or coconut flakes

43. Spirulina Cream of Cauliflower Soup

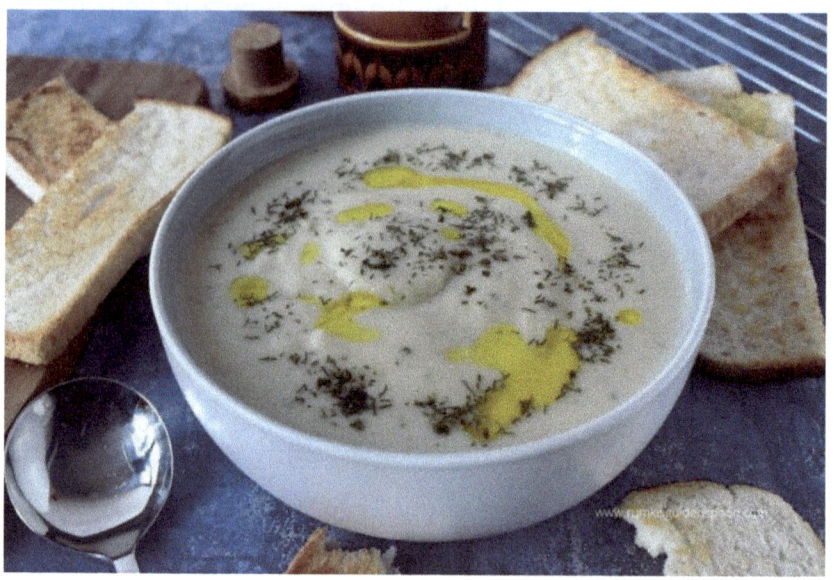

Makes: 2 servings

INGREDIENTS:
- 1 tablespoon sesame, coconut, or grapeseed oil
- ½ yellow onion or fennel bulb
- 2 garlic cloves, minced
- 1 large head of cauliflower, chopped
- 1-quart vegetable broth
- ¼ cup raw, unsalted cashews
- 1 teaspoon blue spirulina
- ½ teaspoons sea salt, plus more to taste
- 2 tablespoons hemp seeds, to garnish

INSTRUCTIONS:
a) In a large pot or Dutch oven, heat oil over medium heat. Add onion and garlic, and sauté for 3 minutes, until slightly brown. Add cauliflower, and sauté for another minute.

b) Add vegetable broth, and increase heat to bring it to a boil. Once boiling, reduce heat and simmer, uncovered, until cauliflower is tender, 20–30 minutes.

c) Remove soup from heat, and cool to a warm room temperature. Transfer soup to a blender with cashews, and blend on high until smooth and creamy, 1 minute. Lastly, add blue spirulina and blend briefly. Stir in salt to taste.

d) Serve topped with hemp seeds.

44. Romanesco creamy soup with kale and spirulina

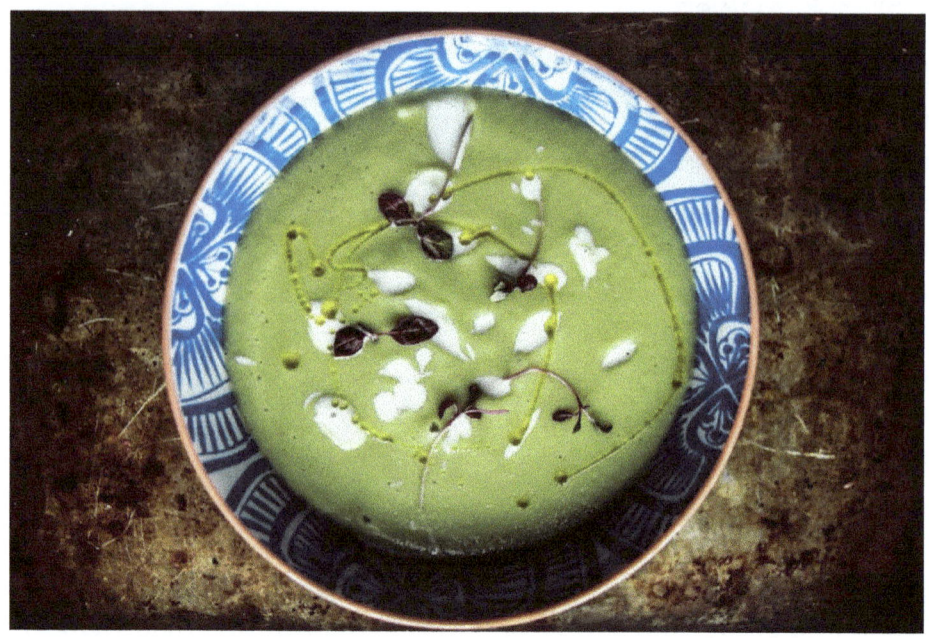

Makes: 4 servings

INGREDIENTS:
- 1 Romanesco
- 2 or 3 green or purple kale leaves
- 1 onion
- 1 garlic clove
- 3 Tbs of oat flakes
- 1 Tbs of powder spirulina
- 2 Tbs of lemon juice
- Lemon zest
- Salt, white pepper, and extra virgin olive oil
- Leek sprouts to decorate and give it a crunchy twist

INSTRUCTIONS
a) Cut the Romanesco in flowers and rinse it gently under the tap with a colander.
b) Take the stem out of the kale leaves and cut them into one-inch pieces.
c) Peel and dice the onion.
d) Smash the garlic clove, peel it and cut it into slices.
e) Sauté the onion until transparent.
f) Add the kale and cook for 3-4 more minutes.
g) Add the Romanesco flowers, and the 3 spoons of oat flakes and add water to cover.
h) Season with salt and pepper and cook for 5 minutes.
i) Set aside from the heat, add the lemon juice and the spirulina powder, and puree until getting a fine consistency.
j) Decorate with leek sprouts and grate the lemon zest over it,

45. Pumpkin and ginger cream soup with spirulina topping

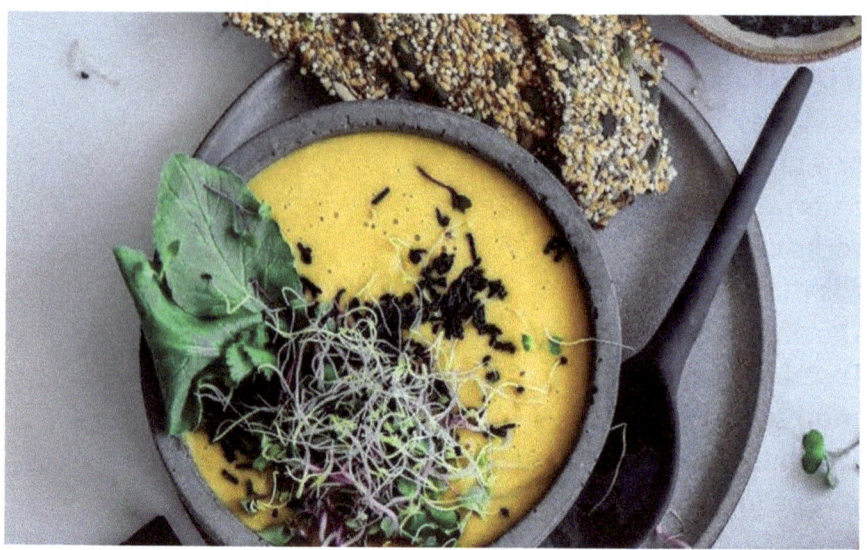

Makes: 2 servings

INGREDIENTS:
- 1 kg pumpkin
- 1 onion
- 1 leek
- 1 slice of ginger
- 1 liter of vegetable stock
- 1 liter of vegetable stock
- 1 teaspoon turmeric
- 1 pinch of pepper
- 1 pinch of salt
- 1 teaspoon spirulina, crunchy

INSTRUCTIONS
a) Chop the onion, leek, and ginger and start frying them in oil.
b) When the ingredients are cooked, add the pumpkin and sauté with the spices: turmeric, salt, and pepper.
c) Add the vegetable stock and cook over medium heat until the pumpkin is cooked, 20 minutes.
d) Mash everything.
e) Serve the toppings: crunchy spirulina, sesame oil, and green leaves.

DESSERT

46. Blue Chia Pudding

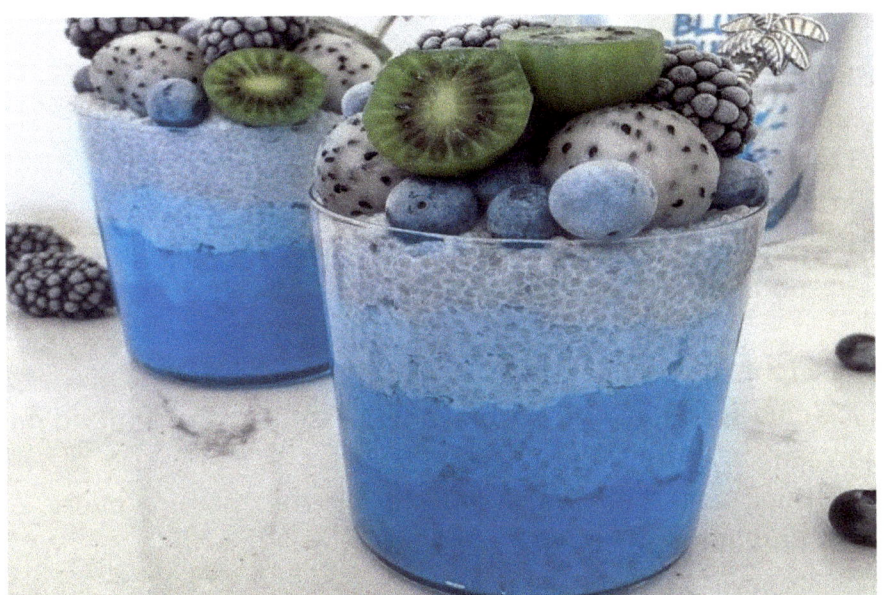

Makes: 2 servings

INGREDIENTS:
- 1 cup of almond milk
- 3.5 tablespoons of white chia seeds
- 1-2 tablespoons of maple syrup
- 1 teaspoon of vanilla essence
- 1 teaspoon Blue Spirulina Powder

INSTRUCTIONS:
a) Place chia seeds, maple syrup, vanilla essence, and almond milk in a jar. Stir
b) everything together, and keep stirring the mixture every 2-3 minutes until it has a jelly-like
c) consistency.
d) In three separate bowls mix 2 tablespoons of coconut yogurt with blue spirulina
e) powder for:
f) The top layer is chia seeds pudding on its own.
g) The lightest blue layer is ⅓ of a teaspoon of blue spirulina powder
h) Middle layer ½ of a teaspoon of blue spirulina powder
i) Darker layer 1 teaspoon of blue spirulina powder
j) Add ¼ of the chia seeds mixture to each blue coconut yogurt and mix through.
k) Layer the jar. Store the jar in the fridge.

47. Spirulina Popsicles

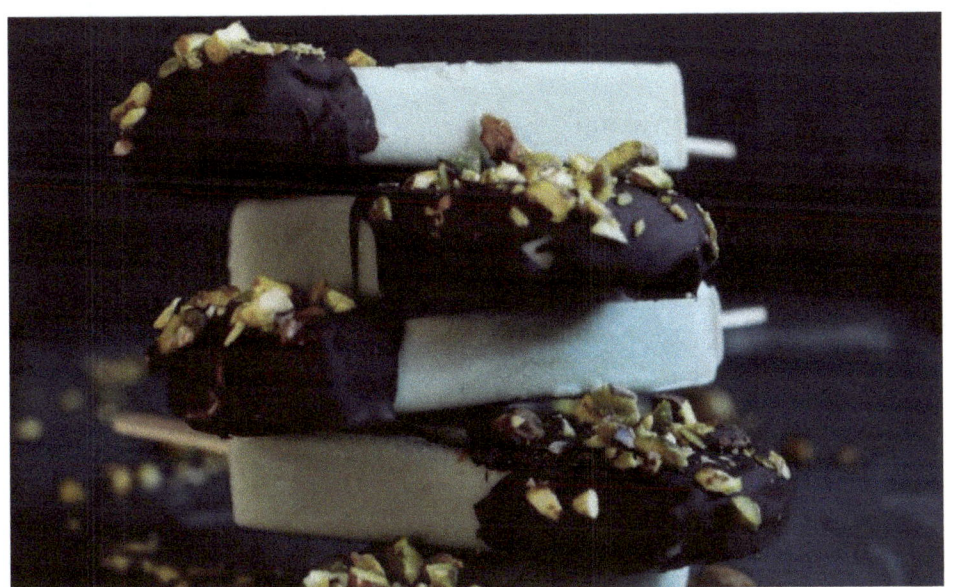

Makes: 8

INGREDIENTS:
- 1 ½ cups dairy-free milk
- 1 cup green grapes
- 2 tablespoons lime juice
- 2 tablespoons maple syrup more or less to taste
- 1 tablespoon green spirulina powder
- 1 tablespoon baobab powder for extra immunity boost of vitamin c and citrus flavor

INSTRUCTIONS:
Stir the spirulina into 2 tablespoons water to dissolve it. Then throw all ingredients in a blender, and blend smoothly.
a) Taste test to be sure the popsicles are not too bitter, yet not too sweet. To sweeten, add more lime juice.
b) Add milk if it is too thick. You want it liquid so the popsicles freeze into icy popsicles.
c) Once adjusted, pour into molds. Put the mold in the freezer for about 30 minutes, then insert the sticks.
d) Freeze the popsicles overnight.
e) To remove from molds without melting pops is always a bit of a challenge, especially with icy pops like these.
f) I run the bottom of the mold under hot water and tug. Keep doing this until I have all the pops out.

48. Coconut Blue Spirulina Raspberry Cheesecake

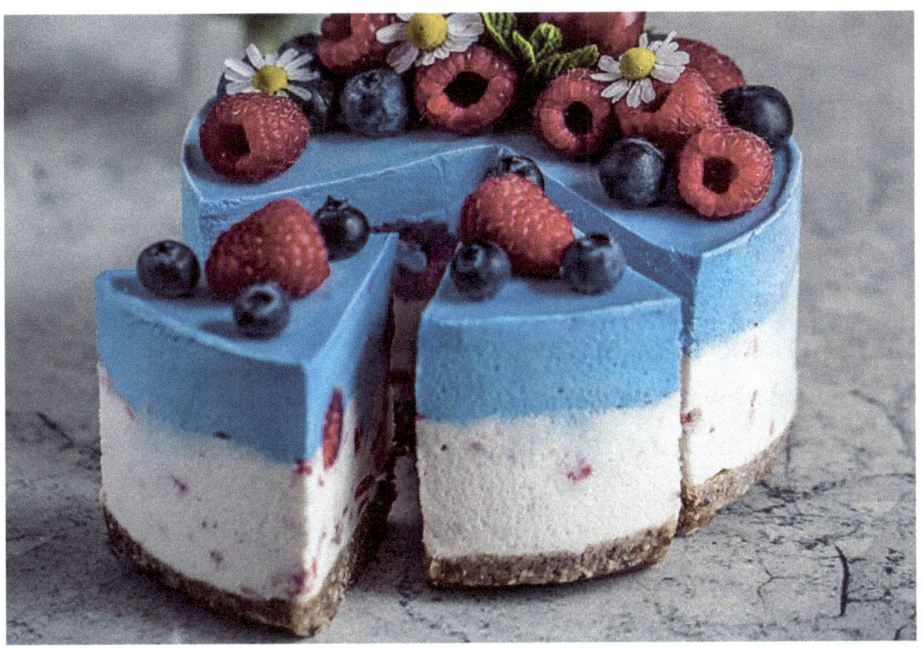

Makes: 6

INGREDIENTS:

CRUST
- 80 g roasted almonds
- 20 g rolled oats ground
- 70 g dates previously soaked in water for a minimum of 1 hour

COCONUT AND RASPBERRY LAYER
- 150 g cashews previously soaked for min 4 hours
- 80 g coconut cream the thickened cream from a can of full-fat coconut milk
- 3-4 tablespoons agave
- 2-3 tablespoons lemon juice
- 2 tablespoons coconut oil
- 20 g shredded coconut
- 15 g dried raspberries chopped
- 100 g fresh raspberries

BLUE SPIRULINA LAYER
- 110 g cashews previously soaked for min 4 hours
- 50 g coconut cream the thickened cream from a can of full-fat coconut milk
- 3 tablespoons agave
- 2 tablespoons coconut oil
- 2-3 tablespoons lemon juice
- 1-2 teaspoons blue spirulina powder

INSTRUCTIONS:

CRUST
a) Line the base of a panettone mold 12x10 cm with baking paper.

b) Place almonds rolled oats, and drained dates into the food processor and process until the mixture sticks together. Adjust sweetness.

c) Once it's all combined and the mixture is nice and sticky, press it evenly onto the bottom of the prepared mold. Place the crust in the fridge while you make the coconut-raspberry layer.

COCONUT AND RASPBERRY LAYER

d) Drain cashews and place them in a blender. Add coconut cream, agave, lemon juice, and coconut oil and blend on high speed until the mixture becomes creamy.

e) Add in 20 g shredded coconut and blend again shortly until all is well combined.

f) Gently fold in fresh and dried raspberries with a spatula.

g) Pour the filling over the crust. Place the cake in the freezer while you make the blue spirulina layer.

BLUE SPIRULINA LAYER

h) Blend cashews, coconut cream, agave, coconut oil, and lemon juice on high speed until the mixture becomes creamy.

i) Add in blue spirulina powder and blend again shortly until you reach the desired color.

j) Carefully pour the mixture on top of the first layer.

k) Place the cake in the freezer to set for at least 4-5 hours.

l) Before serving, top with fresh or frozen berries.

49. Spirulina Ice Cream

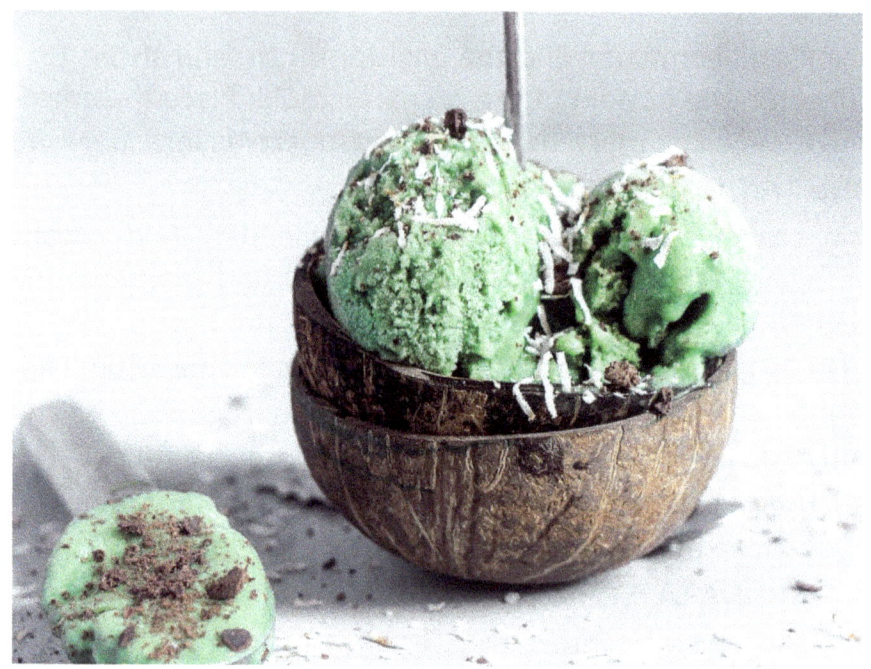

Makes: 2 servings

INGREDIENTS:
- 14 oz full-fat coconut milk
- ¼ cup agave syrup or maple syrup
- 1 teaspoon spirulina
- 1 tablespoon cacao nibs

INSTRUCTIONS:
a) In a blender, mix all the ingredients except the cacao nibs.
b) Transfer the mixture to a bowl. Cover it and place it in the freezer for at least 3-4 hours. Before serving let the mixture thaw for 20 minutes to be able to scoop it out with a medium to large cookie scoop.
c) Sprinkle some cacao nibs on top before serving.

50. Healthy Spirulina Cookies

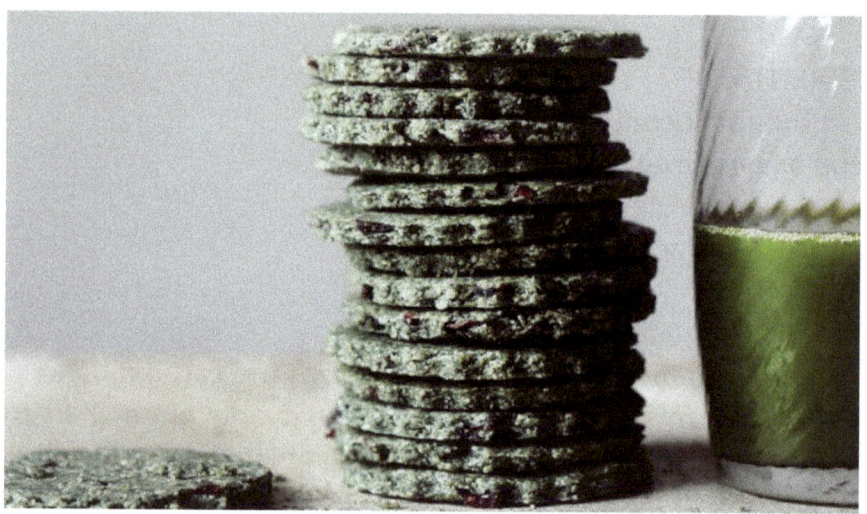

Makes: 8 cookies

INGREDIENTS:
- 1 tablespoon Chia Seeds
- 100 g Vegan Butter
- 50 g White Sugar
- 50 g Brown Sugar
- 1 teaspoon Vanilla Extract
- 100 g gluten-free Flour
- 10 g Corn flour
- ½ teaspoons Baking Soda
- 1.5 tablespoons Spirulina Powder
- ¼ teaspoons Salt
- 50 g White Chocolate or Macadamia Nuts

INSTRUCTIONS:
a) Preheat oven to 200°C / 350°F / 160°C fan.
b) Make a chia egg by adding two and a half tablespoons of hot water to your chia seeds, mix well and set aside.
c) Melt your butter in a saucepan or microwave. Add in the sugar and whisk until smooth.
d) Add the chia egg and vanilla to your butter and sugar and mix well.
e) In a large mixing bowl, sift the flour, cornstarch, baking soda, spirulina, and salt and mix until combined.
f) Pour in the wet mixture and mix well.
g) Fold in your chocolate chunks.
h) Form 8 balls and place them on a cookie sheet lined with parchment paper. Leave around 4cm between each ball.
i) Bake for 10 to 12 minutes until the edges start the crispen.

51. No-Bake Spirulina Cheesecake

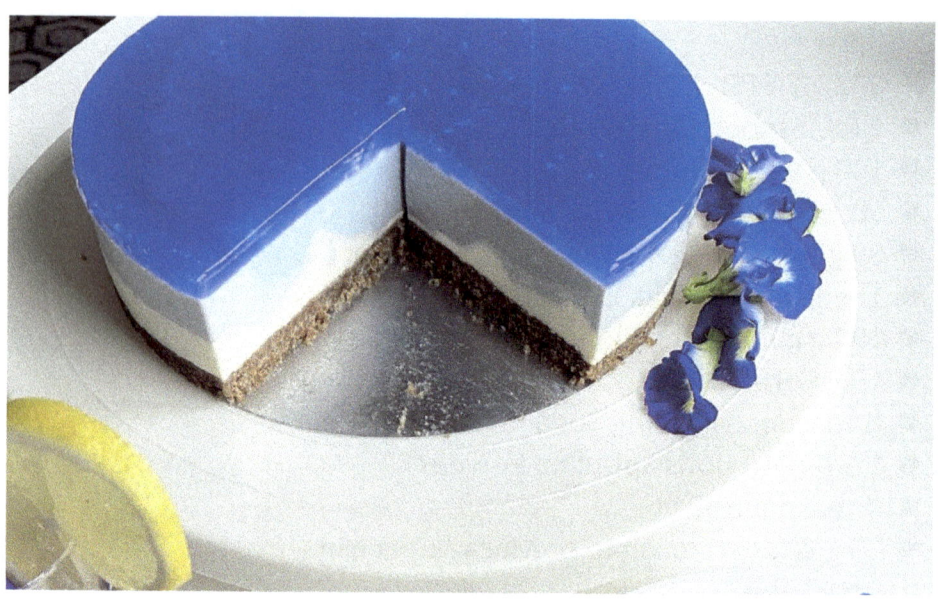

Makes: 6 servings

INGREDIENTS:
- 1 teaspoon Vanilla or Almond Essence

CHEESECAKE FILLING
- 750 g Silken Tofu
- 4 g Agar Agar Powder
- 170 g Sugar-Free Erythritol
- 1.5 teaspoon Spirulina powder

CHEESECAKE BASE
- ½ cup Digestive Biscuits
- 65 mL Coconut Oil, melted

INSTRUCTIONS:
a) To make the cheesecake base, crush the digestive cookies in a plastic food bag using a rolling pin.
b) Then, transfer the cookie crumbs to a bowl, tip in melted coconut oil, and mix well.
c) Transfer the cookie mixture to the cheesecake tin.
d) Press the crumbs firmly with the back of a spoon down into the base to compact them and create an even layer.
e) Then, chill it in the fridge for one hour or freeze it for 30 minutes until the cookie base has set and hardened.
f) Meanwhile, rinse and drain the silken tofu to remove the brine water.
g) Slice the tofu block into cubes, tip them into a food processor, and blitz until smooth and creamy.
h) Transfer the blended tofu into a pot and tip in the agar powder a bit at a time to avoid lumps, stirring until it's incorporated.
i) Then, stir in the sugar or erythritol sweetener for a low-sugar option, followed by the almond or vanilla essence if you're using it.
j) Bring the tofu mixture to a gentle boil and simmer it over low heat for 3 minutes to activate the agar.

k) Stir the mix while it cooks to prevent it from sticking to the bottom of the pan and burning.

l) Next, spoon one-third of the tofu cream over the cold biscuit base.

m) Tap the cake tin on the worktop to remove air bubbles and level the tofu filling with a spatula or the back of a spoon.

n) In a small cup, dissolve the Spirulina powder in little tofu cream until you have no lumps.

o) Then, incorporate the blue pea mix into the remaining two-thirds of the tofu cream.

p) Stir well until you have a uniform blue cheesecake cream.

q) Carefully pour the blue tofu cream over the white tofu layer.

r) Again, tap the cake tin on the worktop to remove air bubbles and level the blue tofu filling with a spatula or the back of a spoon.

s) Wrap the tin with cling film and refrigerate the Spirulina cheesecake for 2-3 hours or until the filling is set.

t) Place the tin on a tall glass, unlock or loosen the cake tin ring, and carefully slide it downward.

u) Once freed, transfer the Spirulina cheesecake onto a serving plate, remove the cake tin base, and garnish the cake to your liking.

52. Spirulina Meringue Baskets

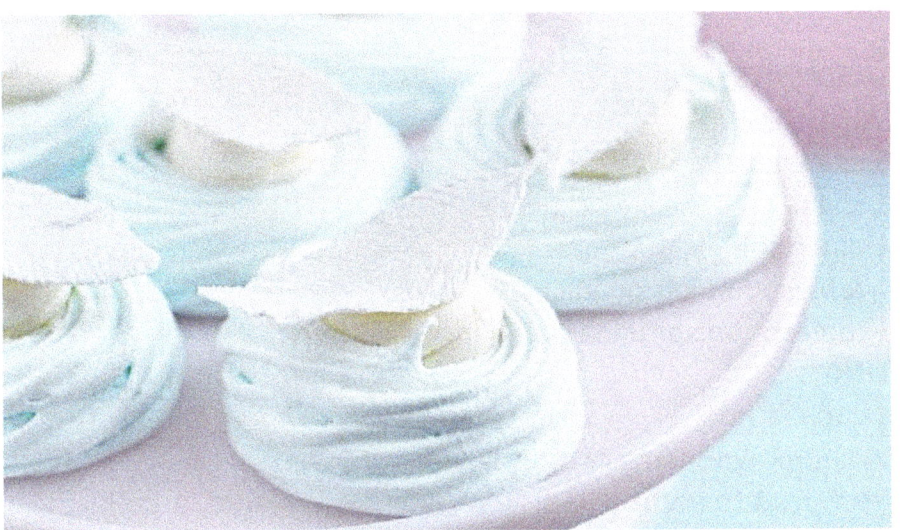

Makes: 11

INGREDIENTS:
MERINGUE
- 3 egg whites
- 1 sugar
- 1 pinch salt
- 1 tablespoon lemon juice
- 1 tablespoon spirulina powder

FILLING
- 1 cup cream
- ¼ cup powder sugar
- fresh fruit to garnish

INSTRUCTIONS

a) To a mixing bowl add egg whites. No egg yolk at all. Meringue doesn't like oils; therefore, any egg yolk or oil residue will affect the outcome.

b) Mix egg whites until white and foamy.

c) Slowly add sugar while continuously mixing the egg whites. White color sugar brings out bright color and gives the meringue firmer texture.

d) Add lemon juice, Spirulina powder and mix until stiff peaks.

e) Transfer the meringue to a piping bag with an open star piping tip. Pipe meringue baskets onto a baking tray lined with silicon mat or parchment paper. Pipe circular base first and three rings on top. Meringue can melt at room temperature so work quickly.

f) Bake the meringue baskets at 210 Fahrenheit for about 3 hours.

g) Check with a toothpick if meringue is dehydrated completely. Toothpick should come out dry and clean.

h) To make the filling, mix cream with powder sugar until stiff.

i) Fill the meringue baskets with the cream and decorate with fresh fruit on top.

53. Spirulina Ice Cream

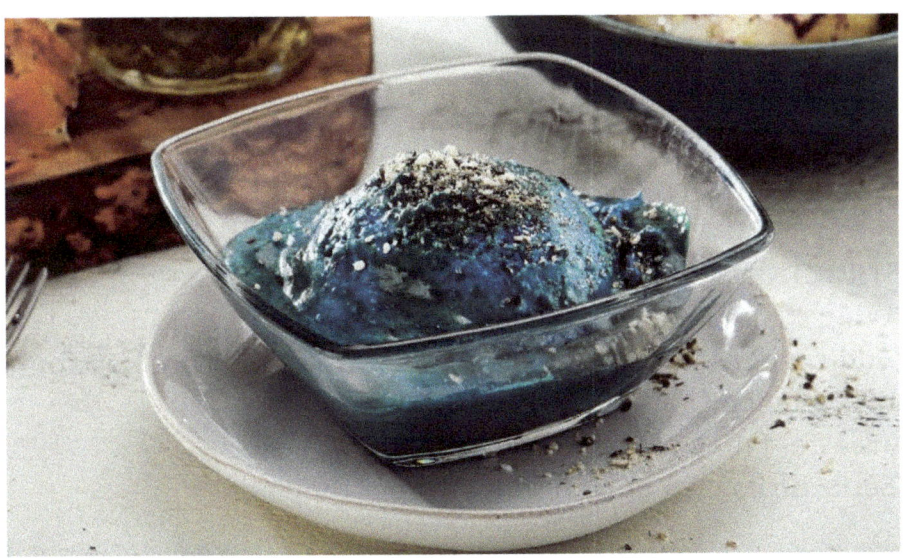

INGREDIENTS:
- 600ml thickened cream
- 1 can condensed milk
- 2 teaspoons spirulina powder

INSTRUCTIONS
a) Whip cream until thickened.
b) Add condensed milk and blue pea powder and continue to mix until combined.
c) Transfer into a container and freeze until solid.
d) Serve on its own or with fruit or other toppings.

54. Spirulina Crepe Cake

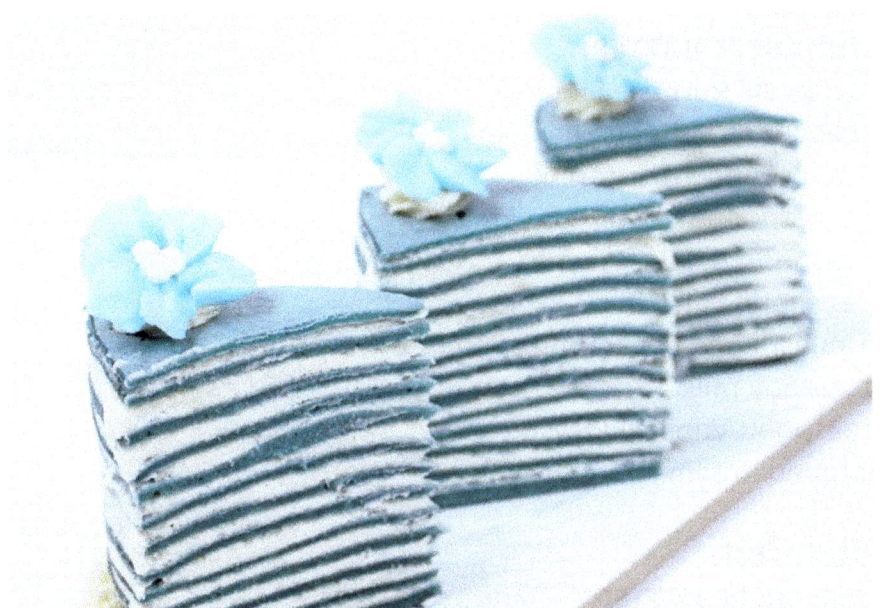

Makes: 12 crepes

INGREDIENTS:
FOR THE CREPE BATTER:
- 1½ cups All Purpose Flour
- 3 teaspoons Spirulina powder
- 1 Tablespoon Cornstarch
- 3 Tablespoons Sugar
- 1 teaspoon Baking Powder
- ¼ teaspoon Salt
- 3 Tablespoons Vegan Butter melted
- 2 cups Soy milk
- 1 teaspoon Vanilla Extract
- Whipped Cream

INSTRUCTIONS:
FOR THE CREPE BATTER:
a) Combine all the ingredients for the crepe batter into a high speed blender or food processor and blend smooth
b) Let it run for 30 seconds and be sure to scrape the sides of the blender carafe for an even mix
c) Pour the batter into a container and refrigerate for at least 1 hour or overnight
d) Stir it vigorously before frying the crepes.
e) With a crepe pan or nonstick 6" diameter frying pan get it hot over a medium to high heat.
f) Lightly spray it with cooking spray and then pour a scant ¼ cup of crepe batter into the hot pan then tilt it all around to get the batter to spread evenly.
g) Cook for approximately 1-2 minutes and then loosen the edges with a small spatula and flip it over carefully to cook on the other side.
h) Be careful not to brown the crepes, you want to keep the vibrant blue color, so you will have to monitor your heat
i) Transfer the cooked crepes to a parchment lined sheet pan

j) Repeat the process until all the crepes are cooked with a very small spray of grease in between each crepe.
k) Layer the crepes on the sheet pan with parchment between each layer do not stack cooked crepe on top of each other without a parchment liner.
l) Once the crepes are cooled you can build the cake with 2 ounces of buttercream or whipped cream between each layer

55. Spirulina Coconut popsicles

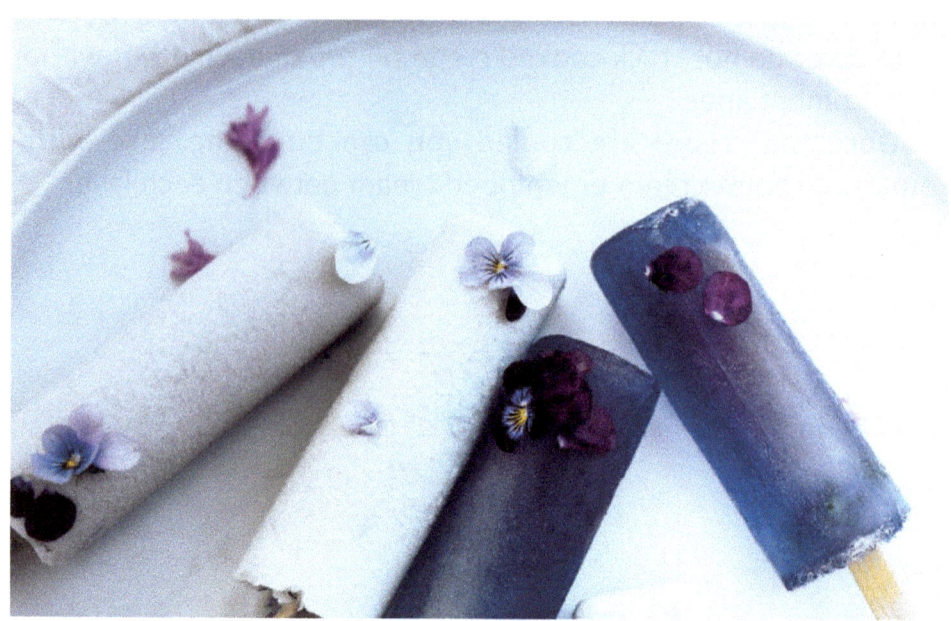

INGREDIENTS:
BLUE POPSICLES:
- 1 cup Spirulina tea
- ¼ cup sake
- sugar to taste

TO BREW BLUE Spirulina TEA:
- 1 TBS blue Spirulina tea
- 1 cup filtered hot water 100°C 3-5 mins
- let it cool to the room temperature

COCONUT:
- 1 can of coconut cream
- 1 seeds of vanilla bean pod
- nigori - unfiltered sake to taste
- maple syrup to taste

INSTRUCTIONS:
a) Mix the blue popsicle ingredients.
b) Mix the coconut popsicle ingredients.
c) Pour mixture into the popsicles molds.
d) Freeze for 8 hours.
e) Run the outside of the molds under running water.
f) Remove the popsicles from the molds.
g) Enjoy!

56. Blueberry Spirulina Parfait

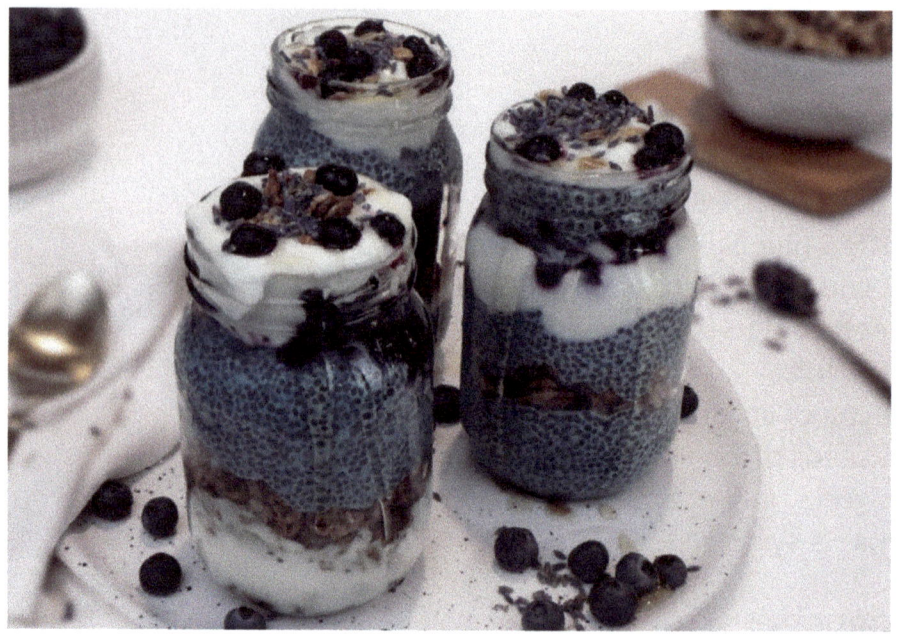

Makes: 1

INGREDIENTS:
- 1 teaspoon Spirulina powder
- ⅔ cup Almond milk
- 3 tablespoons Chia seeds
- 1 teaspoon Maple syrup
- ¼ cup Granola
- ½ cup Vegan Yogurt
- ¼ cup Blueberries

INSTRUCTIONS:
a) In a bowl, whisk together 1 teaspoon Spirulina powder and ⅔ cup almond milk.
b) Mix in 3 tablespoons chia seeds and 1 teaspoon maple syrup and let sit for about 10 minutes.
c) To assemble the parfait, start with chia pudding on the bottom of a glass.
d) Add ¼ cup granola. Add ½ cup plant-based vanilla yogurt.
e) To serve, garnish with ¼ cup blueberries and sprinkle a few extra pieces of granola on top. Enjoy!

57. Spirulina Pandan Cake

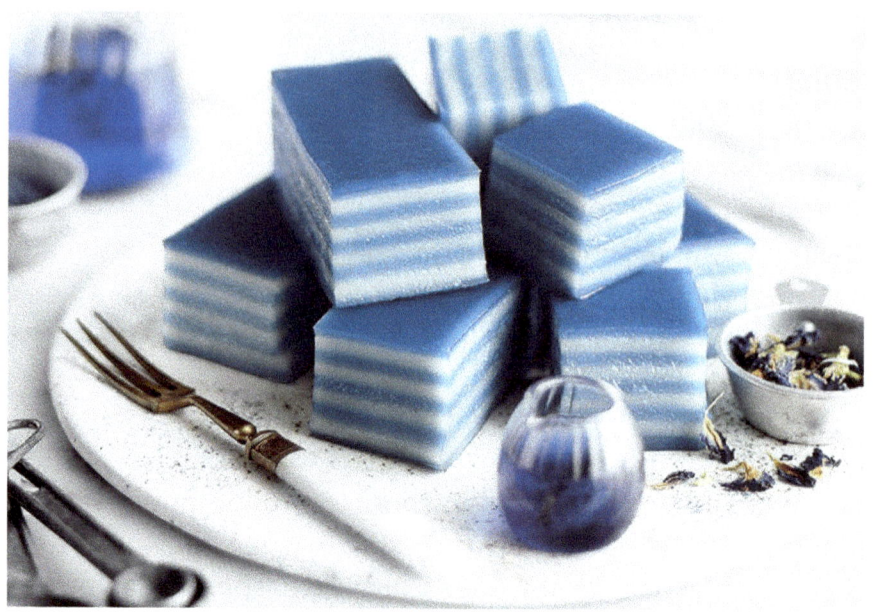

INGREDIENTS:
- 1 ½ cups water
- 2 ½ cups coconut milk
- 3 pandan leaves, knotted
- 1 ½ Emerald Pandan Leaf Powder
- ¾ cup sugar of choice
- ½ teaspoon salt
- 2 cups tapioca flour
- ¾ cup rice flour
- ¾ cup regular flour
- 2 teaspoon Spirulina powder dissolved in 2 teaspoon water

INSTRUCTIONS:
a) In a large pot combine water, coconut milk, sugar, salt, pandan leaves, and Emerald Pandan Leaf Powder together till sugar dissolved. Turn off heat, allow mixture to cool completely.
b) In a mixing bowl mix together tapioca flour, rice flour and regular flour. Set aside.
c) Discard pandan leaves from the coconut milk mixture. Gradually add coconut mixture into the dry mixture with a hand whisk. Whisk until smooth and combine. Then strain mixture through a sieve.
d) Divide mixture in two equal portions, add dissolved Spirulina powder into one portion, keeping one portion white.
e) Line a cake pan with parchment paper then place it in the steamer.
f) Use same size measuring cups to spoon the mixtures.
g) Start with blue color, then white and blue. Pour ½ cup blue batter into the pan. Steam for 5 minutes.
h) Then pour in white layer and steam for 5 minutes. Repeat this sequence until you get 9 layers. Lastly, steam for 15 minutes.
i) Let it cool for at least 4 hours before slicing. Use an oiled knife to slice cake and enjoy!

58. Spirulina Marble Bundt

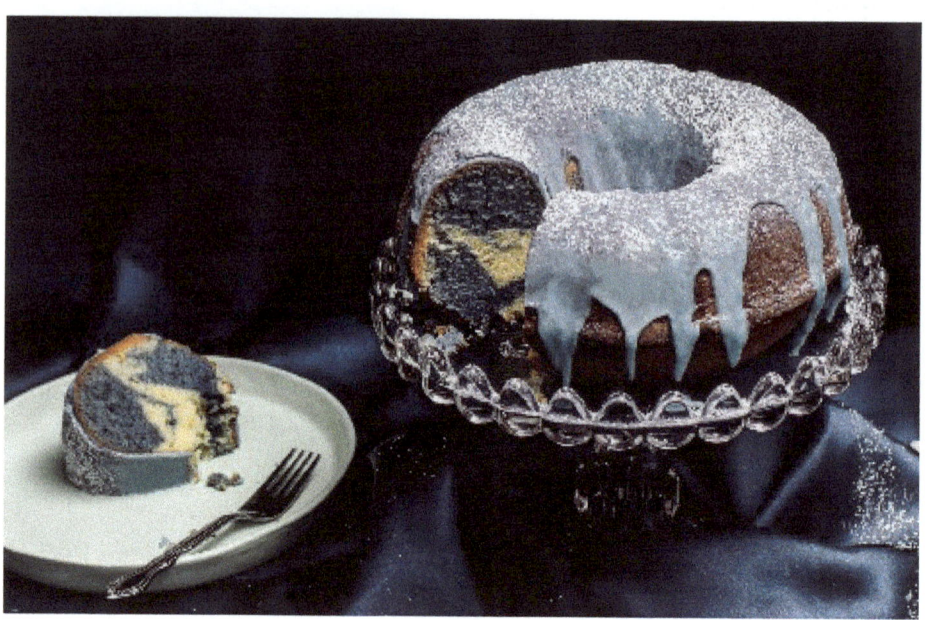

Makes: 1 Bundt

INGREDIENTS
Spirulina powder MARBLE BUNDT
- 3½ cups all-purpose flour
- 4 teaspoons baking powder
- ¾ teaspoons salt
- ¾ cup unsalted butter room temperature
- ½ cup vegetable oil
- 1¾ cups granulated sugar
- 3 eggs + 2 egg whites room temperature
- 4 teaspoons vanilla
- 1½ cups buttermilk
- 1 tablespoon Spirulina powder
- 1 tablespoon milk

VANILLA GLAZE
- 1½ cups powdered sugar
- 1 teaspoon Spirulina powder
- ½ teaspoon vanilla
- 2-4 tablespoons milk

INSTRUCTIONS
Spirulina powder MARBLE BUNDT
a) Preheat the oven to 350°F / 175°C. Butter and generously flour a 12 cup capacity Bundt pan.
b) In a medium sized bowl, whisk together the flour, baking powder, and salt. Set aside.
c) In the bowl of a stand mixer fitted with the paddle attachment, beat together the butter, oil, and sugar for 5 minutes until light and fluffy.
d) Scrape down the sides of the bowl, and add in one egg at a time, beating for 20 seconds between each addition. Add in the vanilla with the last egg.
e) Alternate between adding the flour mixture and the buttermilk. Fold in ⅓ of the flour mixture, then ½ of the buttermilk, ⅓ of the

flour, the remaining ½ of the buttermilk, and the remaining ⅓ of the flour.

f) Remove ~3 cups of batter and place it into a medium sized bowl. In a small bowl, mix together the Spirulina powder and milk. To the 3 cups, gently mix in the Spirulina powder mixture until the batter is completely blue.

g) Evenly spread ~⅓ of the vanilla batter into the Bundt. Use ~⅓ of the blue batter to place big dollops over the vanilla, then use a knife to gently swirl the blue around.

h) Add another ⅓ of the vanilla on top, repeat the dollops and swirling two times, ending with the blue batter on top.

i) Bake for 50-60 minutes, until a knife inserted in the Bundt comes out clean or with only a few moist crumbs.

j) Let the cake cool in the pan for 10-15 minutes. Once the pan is cool enough to touch, flip the cake out onto a clean surface. Let the cake cool completely before frosting.

VANILLA GLAZE

k) In a bowl, mix together all of the ingredients starting with 2 tablespoons of milk. Add more milk as needed to get to your desired consistency.

l) Pour the glaze evenly over the cake.

m) Optional: Pour 1 teaspoon of white food dye into a bowl. Use a paintbrush to speckle the cake. Top with rose petals and white sugar pearl sprinkles.

n) Serve, and enjoy!

59. Banana Spirulina Nice Cream

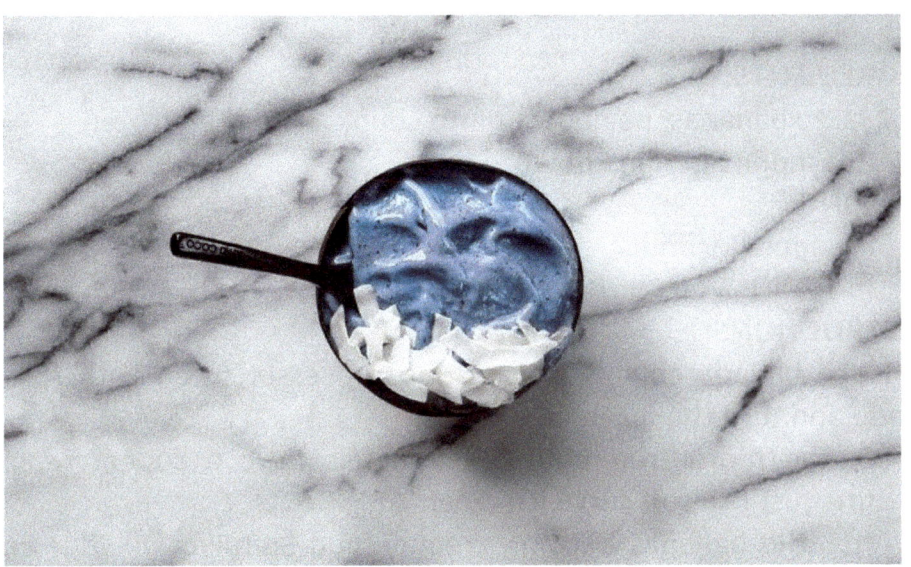

Makes: 2-3 servings

INGREDIENTS:
- 2 large bananas, peeled, cut into chunks, and then frozen
- 1 teaspoon Spirulina powder

TOPPING:
- Shredded Coconut

INSTRUCTIONS:
a) Place banana chunks into a food processor fitted with the S blade and turn the machine on.
b) Let the motor run until the bananas have a super creamy texture, just like soft serve ice cream.
c) After the bananas become creamy, add Spirulina powder and blend.
d) Serve immediately with shredded coconut.

60. Spirulina and Raspberry Friands

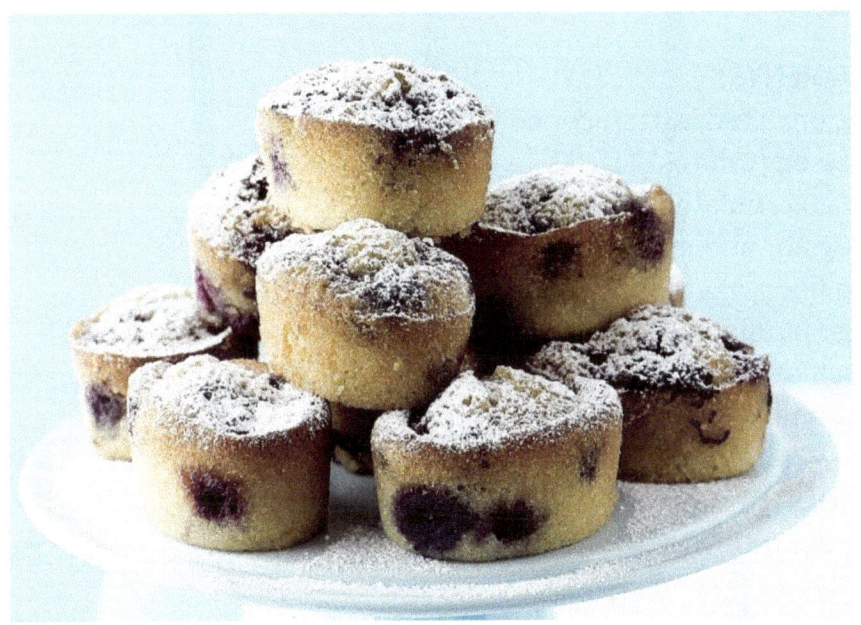

Makes: 4

INGREDIENTS:
- 95g unsalted butter, cubed
- 135g egg whites
- 150g granulated sugar
- 100g almond meal
- 60g flour
- 12g Spirulina powder
- pinch of salt
- Optional: Fresh/frozen raspberries

INSTRUCTIONS:
a) Grease your muffin tins thoroughly with butter and dust flour sparingly over them.
b) Heat the butter in a pan over the low-medium fire and allow it to cook until it is golden brown.
c) Turn off the fire and take it off the heat once it is golden brown, otherwise, it will go from golden brown to black very quickly.
d) Allow cooling to room temperature while you prepare the rest of the ingredients.
e) In a bowl, place sugar, flour and ground almond, Spirulina powder, and salt together.
f) Whisk the dry ingredients a little.
g) Add in the butter and whisk to combine.
h) Add in the egg whites slowly while whisking till incorporated. You do not need to create too much volume in the egg whites. I do all this by hand as you just need the batter to come together.
i) Spoon the friands batter into the greased muffin molds. Place a raspberry into the center of the friand. Bake in a 190 degrees preheated oven for about 15 minutes, or until it springs back to touch.
j) Allow it to cool slightly in the muffin tins before unmolding. Cool them completely on wire racks before serving.

61. Spirulina Truffles

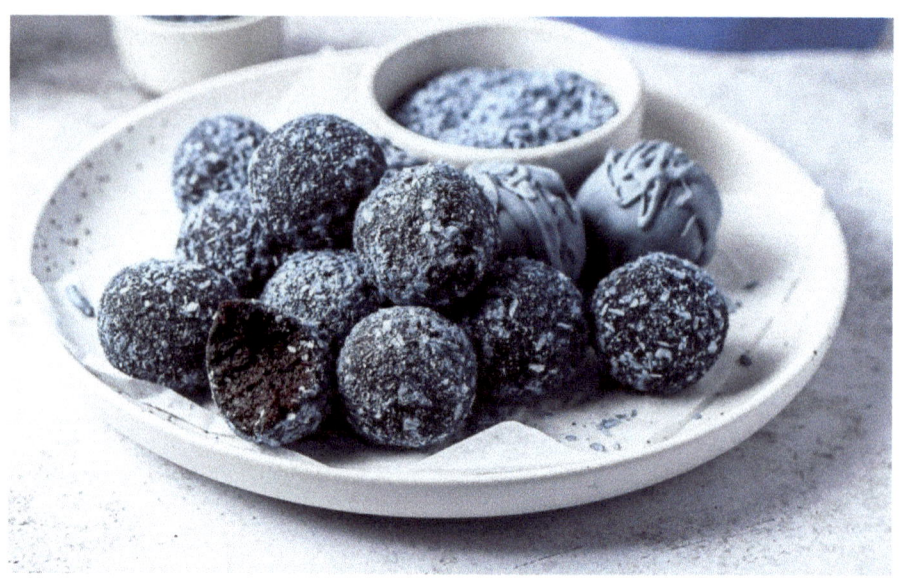

Makes: about 50 truffles

INGREDIENTS:
- 225 grams of heavy cream
- ¼ cup maple syrup
- 2 tablespoons brown sugar
- 1 tablespoon Spirulina, plus another tablespoon for dusting
- 340 grams bittersweet chocolate, chopped finely
- Pinch of kosher salt

INSTRUCTIONS:
a) Bring cream to a simmer in a small saucepan over a gentle heat, add the maple syrup and brown sugar, and stir until dissolved, about 2 minutes.
b) Add 1 tablespoon of Spirulina, stir until dissolved, and set aside.
c) Place the chocolate in a large mixing bowl and pour in the cream mixture. Mix thoroughly, and pour into a baking sheet lined with parchment paper. Smooth it out with a rubber spatula.
d) Cool in the refrigerator for about an hour.
e) Using a spoon, scoop out a heaping teaspoon, and make a ball using the palms of your hands.
f) Repeat until all the chocolate is used –you should wind up with about 50 truffles.
g) Line them up on a tray or plate, and dust them with the additional Spirulina, using a fine sieve.
h) Top with a very light sprinkling of Spirulina.

62. Spirulina Tea Fudge

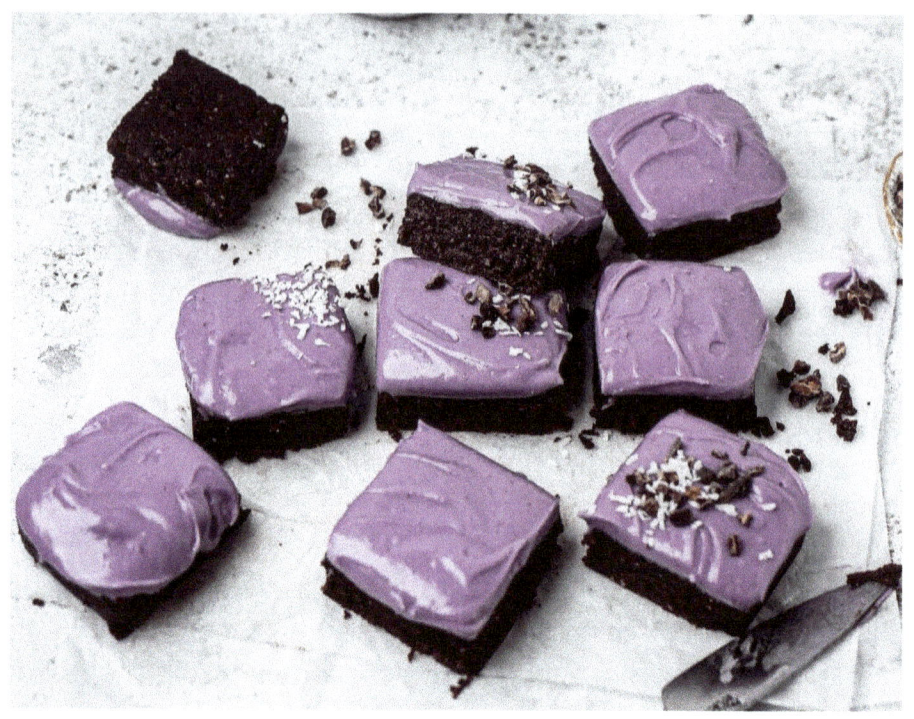

Makes: 4

INGREDIENTS:
- 85 g Roasted almond butter
- 60 g Oat flour
- 1 cup Unsweetened vanilla almond milk
- 168 g protein powder
- 4 ounces Dark chocolate, melted
- 4 teaspoons Spirulina powder
- 1 teaspoon stevia extract
- 10 drops Lemon

INSTRUCTIONS:
a) Melt butter in a saucepan and add oats flour, Spirulina, protein powder, lemon drops, and stevia. Mix well.
b) Now pour milk and stir constantly until well combined.
c) Transfer the mixture to a loaf pan and refrigerate until set.
d) Drizzle melted chocolate on top and refrigerate again until the chocolate is firm.
e) Slice into 5 bars and enjoy.

63. Spirulina Pumpkin Cream

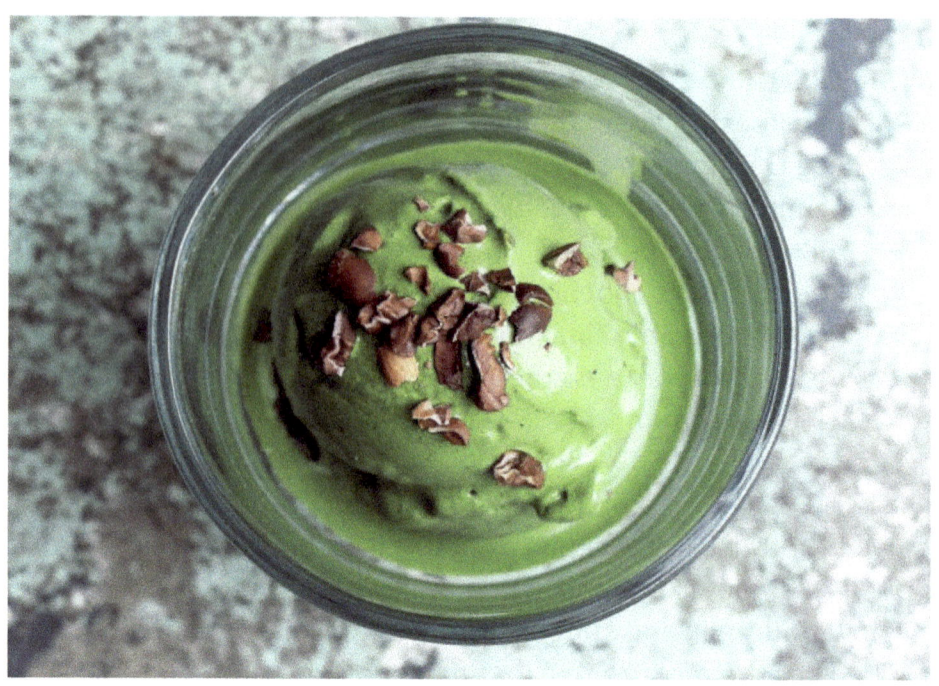

Makes: 2

INGREDIENTS:
- 1 can frozen canned pumpkin
- Coconut water
- 2 Dates
- 1 Tablespoon Spirulina powder

INSTRUCTIONS:
a) Place all ingredients through your food processor
b) Serve in a pretty bowl
c) Decorate with the topping of your choice.

64. Avocado Spirulina Nice Cream

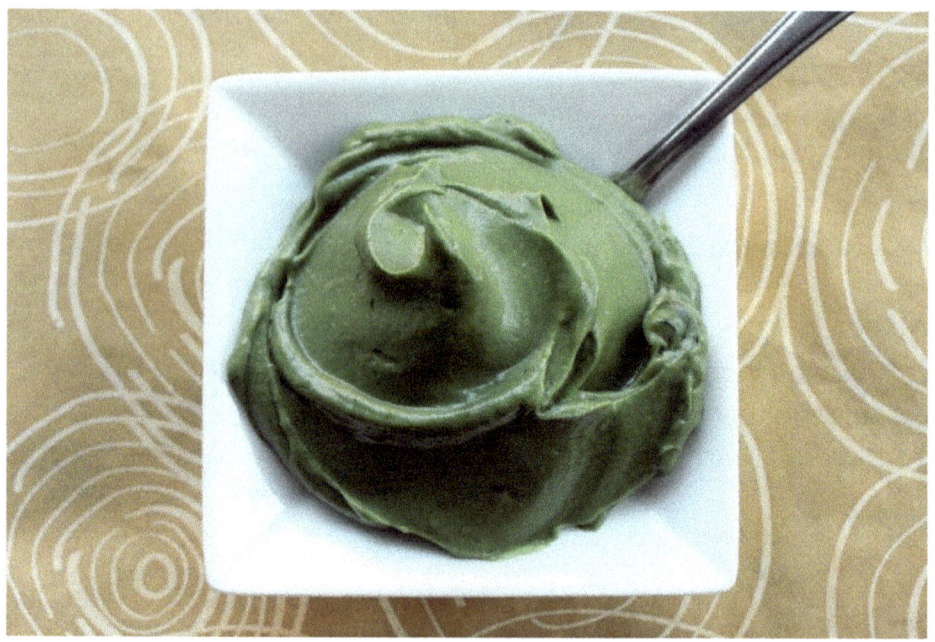

Makes: 2-3 servings

INGREDIENTS:
- 2 avocados, peeled, sliced and frozen
- 1 teaspoon Spirulina powder

INSTRUCTIONS:
a) Mash avocado until you have a super creamy texture, just like soft serve ice cream.
b) Add Spirulina powder and blend.
c) Serve immediately.

65. Spirulina Berry Cups

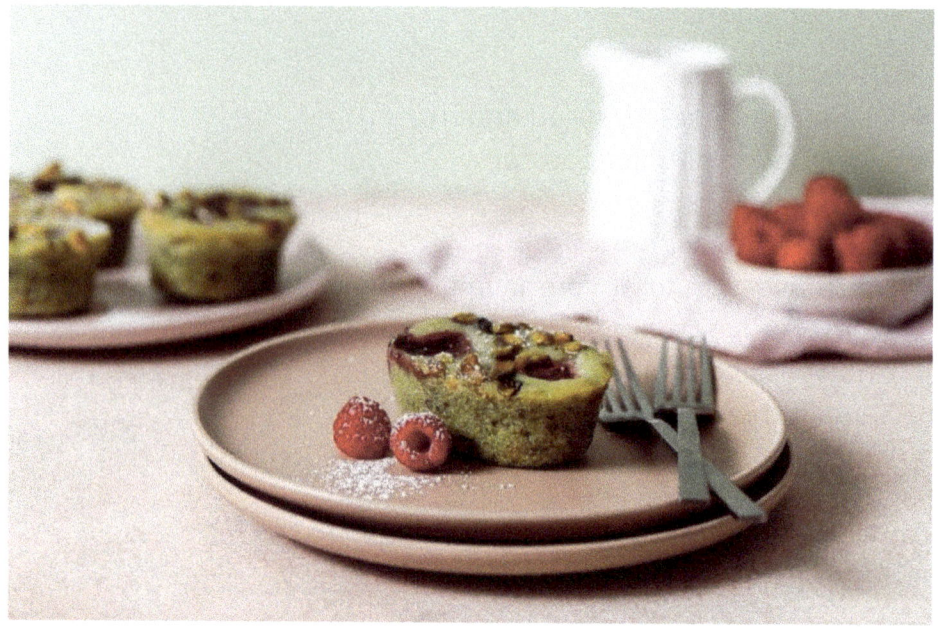

Makes: 4

INGREDIENTS:
- 95g unsalted butter, cubed
- 135g egg whites
- 150g granulated sugar
- 100g almond meal
- 60g chickpea flour
- 12g Spirulina
- pinch of salt
- Berries

INSTRUCTIONS:
k) Grease your muffin tins with butter and dust flour over them.
l) Heat the butter in a pan over the low-medium fire.
m) Turn off the fire and take it off the heat once it is golden brown.
n) In a bowl, place sugar, chickpea flour and ground almond, Spirulina powder, and salt together.
o) Whisk the dry ingredients a little.
p) Add in the butter and whisk to combine.
q) Add in the egg whites slowly while whisking till incorporated.
r) Spoon the batter into the greased muffin molds.
s) Place a berry into the center.
t) Bake in a 190 degrees preheated oven for about 15 minutes, or until it springs back to touch.
u) Allow it to cool slightly in the muffin tins before unmolding.
v) Cool them completely on wire racks before serving.

66. Spirulina Coconut balls

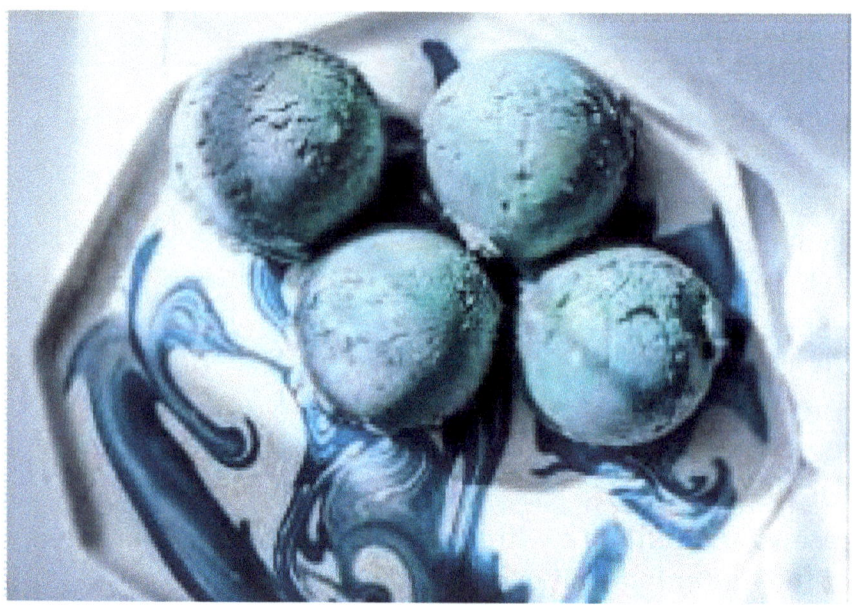

Makes: 50

INGREDIENTS:
- 225 grams of coconut cream
- ¼ cup maple syrup
- 2 tablespoons brown sugar
- 1 tablespoon Spirulina, plus another tablespoon for dusting
- 340 grams bittersweet chocolate, chopped finely
- Salt or kosher salt

INSTRUCTIONS:
i) Bring cream to a simmer in a small saucepan over a gentle heat, add the maple syrup and brown sugar, and stir until dissolved, about 2 minutes.
j) Add 1 tablespoon of Spirulina, stir until dissolved, and set aside.
k) Place the chocolate in a large mixing bowl and pour in the cream mixture.
l) Mix thoroughly, and pour into a baking sheet lined with parchment paper. Smooth it out with a rubber spatula.
m) Cool in the refrigerator for about an hour.
n) Using a spoon, scoop out a heaping teaspoon, and make a ball using the palms of your hands.
o) Line them up on a tray or plate, and dust them with the additional Spirulina, using a fine sieve.

AUCES

67. Spirulina Hummus

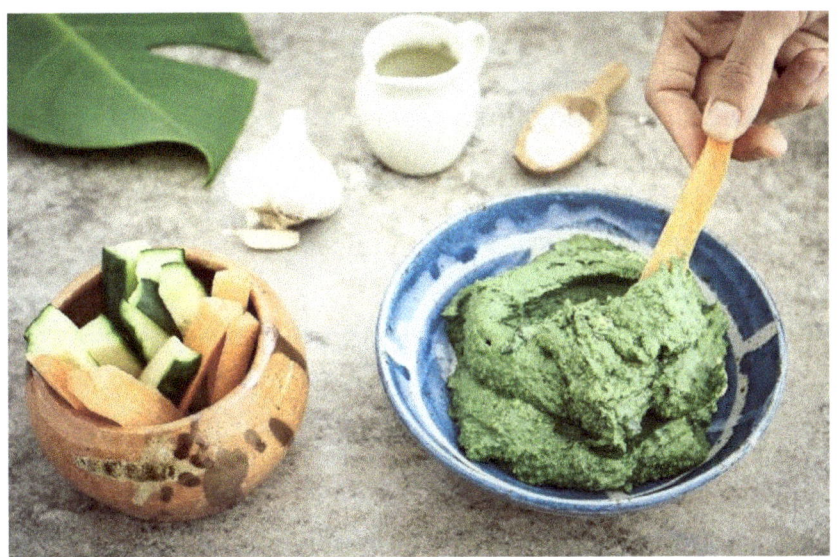

Makes: 2 servings

INGREDIENTS:
- 1 can chickpeas, drained, liquid reserved
- 1 tablespoon olive oil
- 2 teaspoons tahini
- 1 tablespoon freshly pressed lemon juice
- 1 clove garlic, crushed
- ½ teaspoon salt

INSTRUCTIONS:
a) Place the chickpeas, olive oil, tahini, lemon juice, garlic, and salt in a food processor.
b) Turn on the food processor and slowly pour in some of the reserved chickpea liquid while the machine runs.
c) When the mixture is fully combined and smooth, transfer it into a serving dish.

68. Spirulina Guacamole Dip

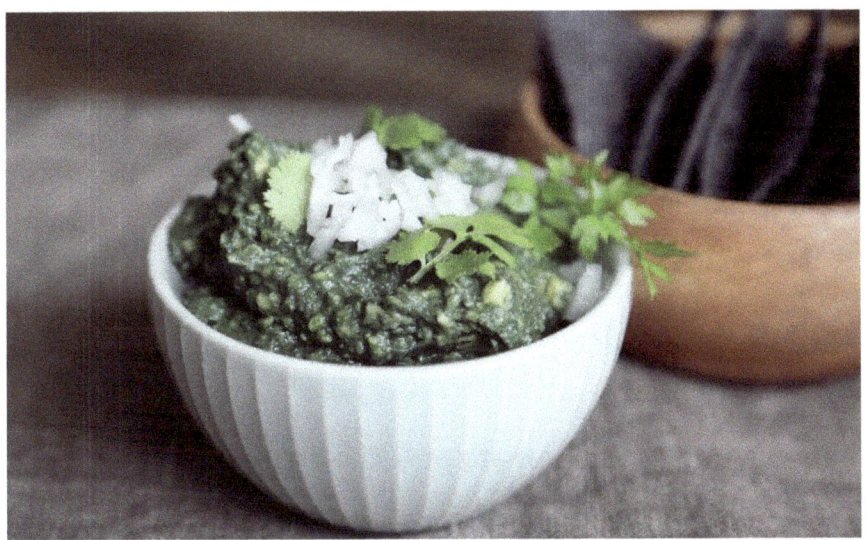

Makes: 2 servings

INGREDIENTS:
- 2 avocados, pitted
- Juice of 1 lemon
- Juice of 1 lime
- 1 clove garlic, roughly chopped
- 1 medium yellow onion, roughly chopped
- 1 jalapeno, sliced
- 1 cup cilantro leaves
- 3 tablespoons spirulina
- 1 seeded and chopped tomato or ½ cup grape tomatoes, halved
- Salt and pepper to taste

INSTRUCTIONS:
a) Put all ingredients, except for tomatoes, into a blender and mix until combined.
b) Stir in tomatoes and season to taste.

69. Spirulina Pesto

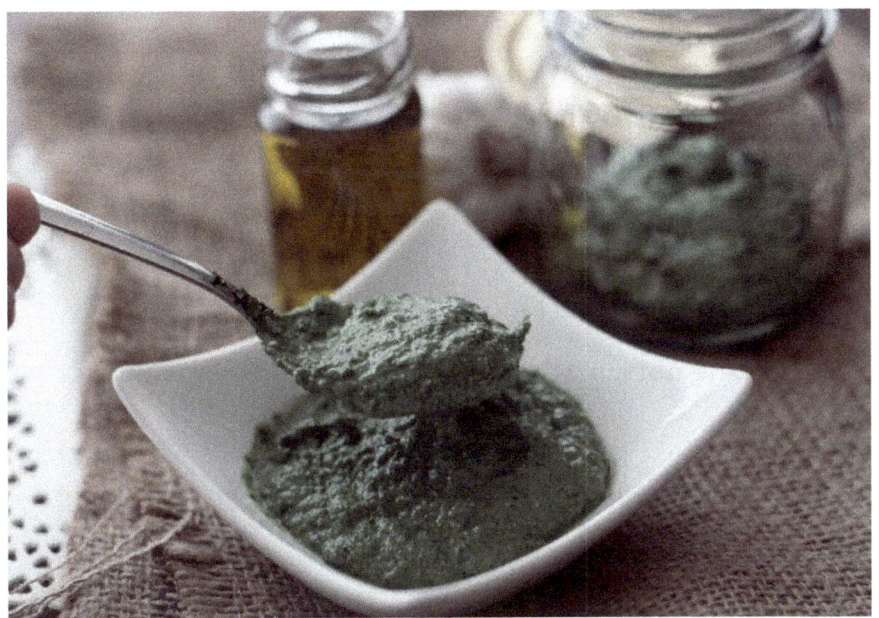

Makes: 2 servings

INGREDIENTS:
- 1 packed cup of fresh basil leaves
- 3-5 tablespoons virgin olive oil
- 2 tablespoons parmesan cheese
- 3 cloves garlic
- 2 teaspoons Spirulina
- Pinch of salt
- 2 ounces pine nuts, macadamia nuts, almonds, or walnuts

INSTRUCTIONS:
a) Blend all ingredients.

70. Spirulina Paté

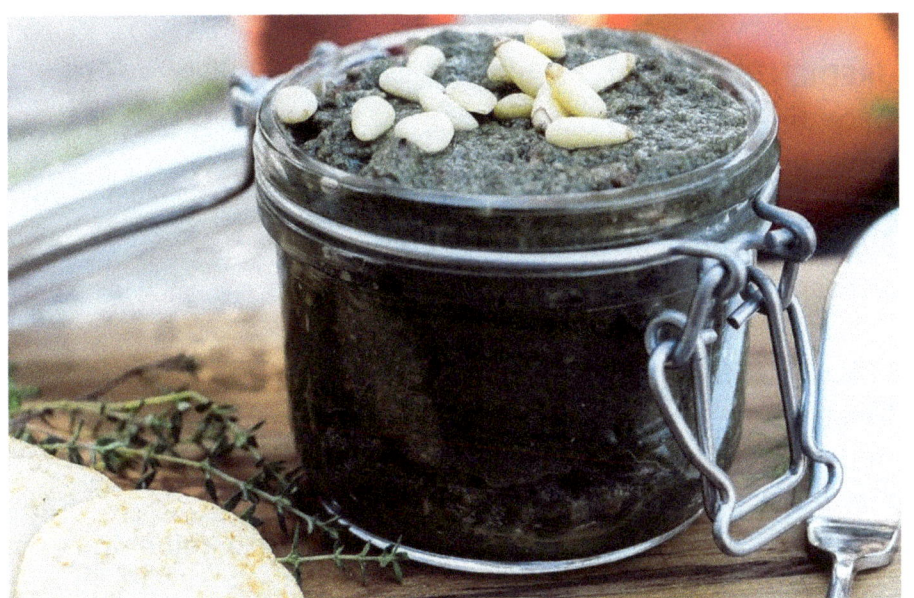

Makes: 2 servings

INGREDIENTS:
- Juice of half lemon
- 1 teaspoon soy sauce
- 1 tablespoon olive oil
- 1 clove crushed garlic
- 1 teaspoon Spirulina

INSTRUCTIONS:
a) Mix the Spirulina with the garlic.
b) Add the lemon juice and soy sauce, and mix well with a fork. Stir in the olive oil.
c) Serve on toast or crackers with slices of tomato and onion.

71. Fresh Salsa and Spirulina

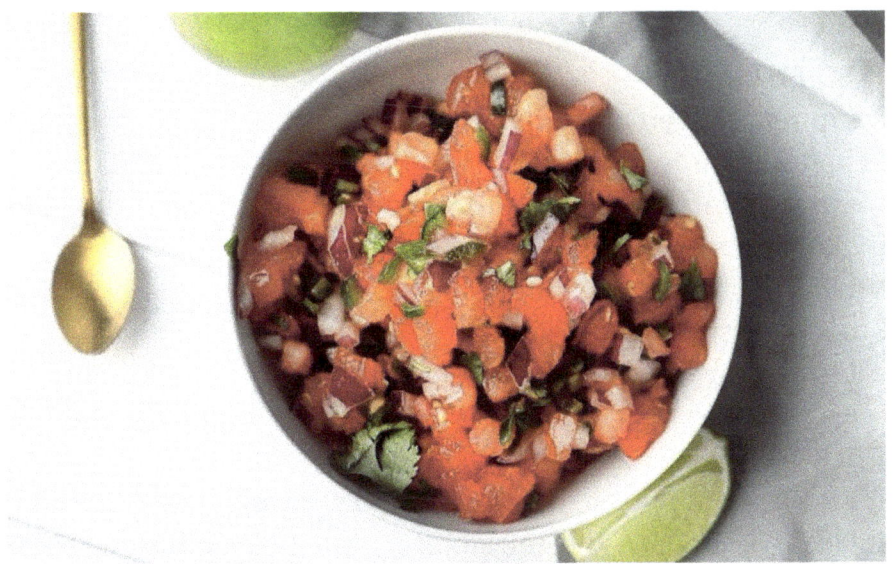

Makes: 2 servings

INGREDIENTS:
- ½ cup finely diced onion
- 2 cloves of garlic, minced
- 3 Roma tomatoes, peel and remove the seeds. sliced
- 1-2 chili peppers, choose your favorite kind.
- A handful of chopped fresh cilantro
- 1 to 2 tablespoons lime juice
- salt and pepper

INSTRUCTIONS:
a) In a bowl, combine all ingredients and stir well.
b) Chill for 2 hours in the refrigerator, for flavor infusion, before serving.

72. Spirulina Salad Dressing

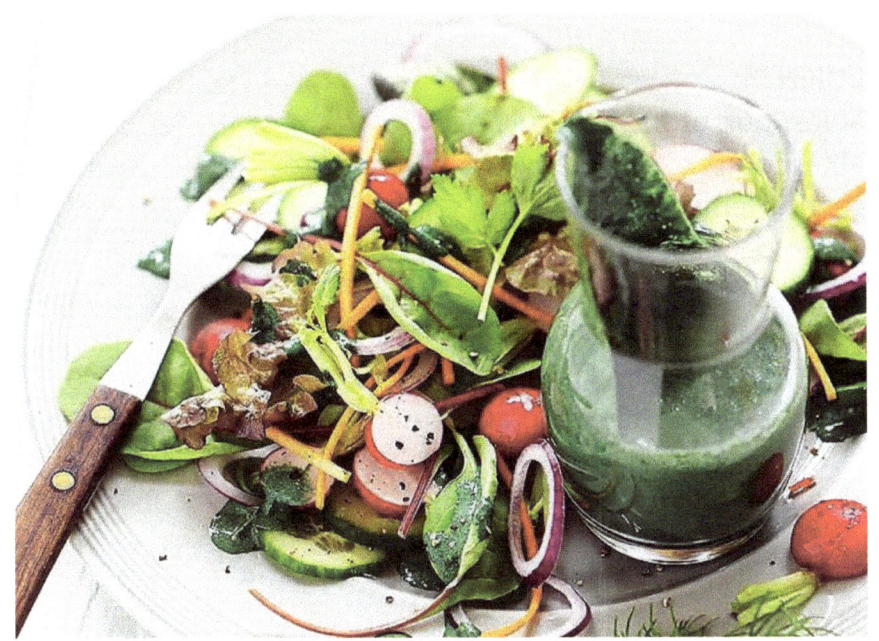

Makes: 2 servings

INGREDIENTS:
- 1 tablespoon of fresh Spirulina
- 2 tablespoons of olive oil
- Juice of ½ lemon
- cayenne pepper to taste

INSTRUCTIONS:
a) Put all the ingredients together and mix.
b) Choose your favorite salad and pour the Spirulina dressing over it.

SMOOTHIES AND COCKTAILS

73. **Mermaid Lemonade**

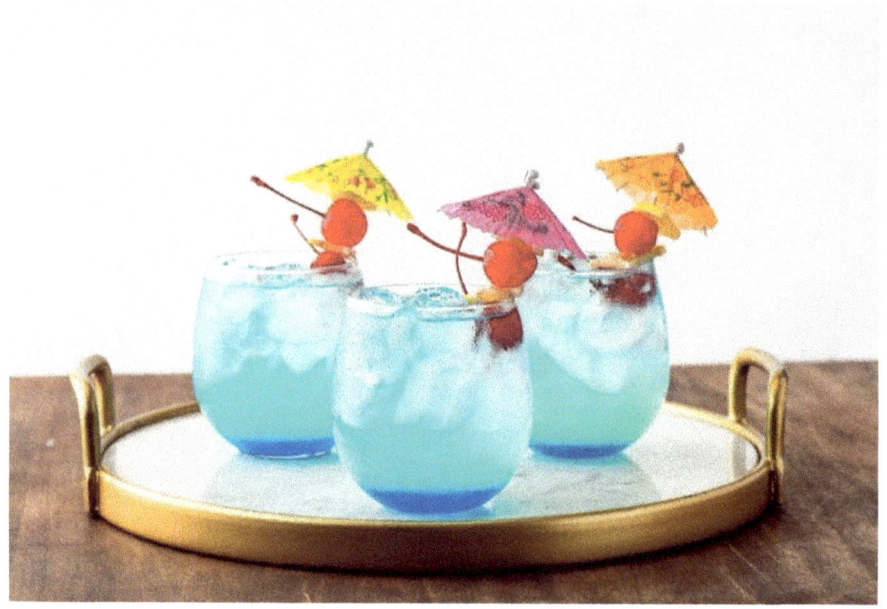

Makes: 5-6 cups

INGREDIENTS:
- 4 cups Water
- 4 large Lemons, squeezed
- ½ cup Agave Nectar
- 1 teaspoon E3 Live Blue Spirulina
- 1 pinch Salt

INSTRUCTIONS:
a) Wash the lemons and cut them in half. Using a citrus press or your hands, squeeze the lemon juice into a bowl, removing any seeds. You should get about 1 cup of fresh lemon juice.
b) Whisk together the agave nectar with the lemon juice until thoroughly combined.
c) In a large pitcher, combine the water, agave/lemon juice, blue spirulina, and a pinch of salt. Stir until well combined and the spirulina powder has dissolved.
d) Refrigerate or pour over ice and enjoy!

74. Blue Smoothie Bowl

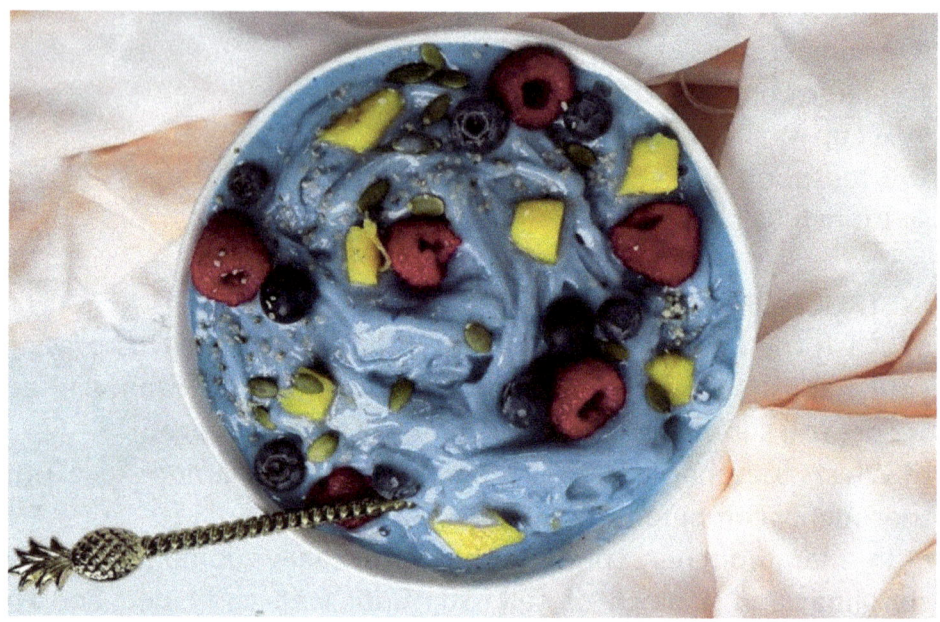

Makes: 1 smoothie bowl

INGREDIENTS:
- 1 ½ ripe bananas, peeled and frozen
- 1 cup fresh mango, frozen
- ½ cup coconut milk yogurt
- ¼ cup unsweetened almond milk, or coconut milk
- ¼ cup orange juice
- 1 teaspoon lime zest
- 2 to 3 teaspoons blue spirulina powder, or blue pea flower powder
- ½ cup ice

TOPPINGS:
- ⅓ cup Bob's Red Mill Paleo Muesli
- ¼ cup fresh blueberries
- 1 Kiwi, peeled and sliced
- ¼ cup fresh mango, peeled and chopped

INSTRUCTIONS:
a) Add all ingredients for the smoothie bowl to a blender and blend until smooth.
b) Pour blue smoothie into a bowl and top with paleo muesli and fresh fruit.

75. Ginger Lemonade with Blue Spirulina

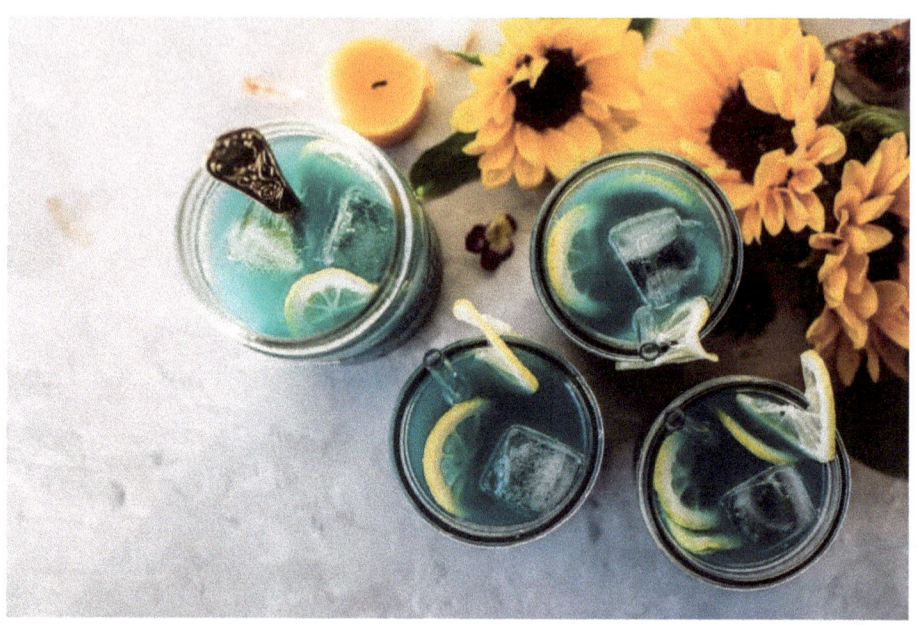

Makes: 4-6 Servings

INGREDIENTS:
- 2 cups of filtered water
- 1 cup of ginger tea
- 2-4 lemons
- 1 scoop of spirulina
- stevia to taste
- 1 cup of ice

INSTRUCTIONS:
a) Brew your ginger tea.
b) Add water, lemon juice, blue milk, sweetener, and CBD oil.
c) Add ice & enjoy!

76. Coconut Tequila Kefir Cocktail

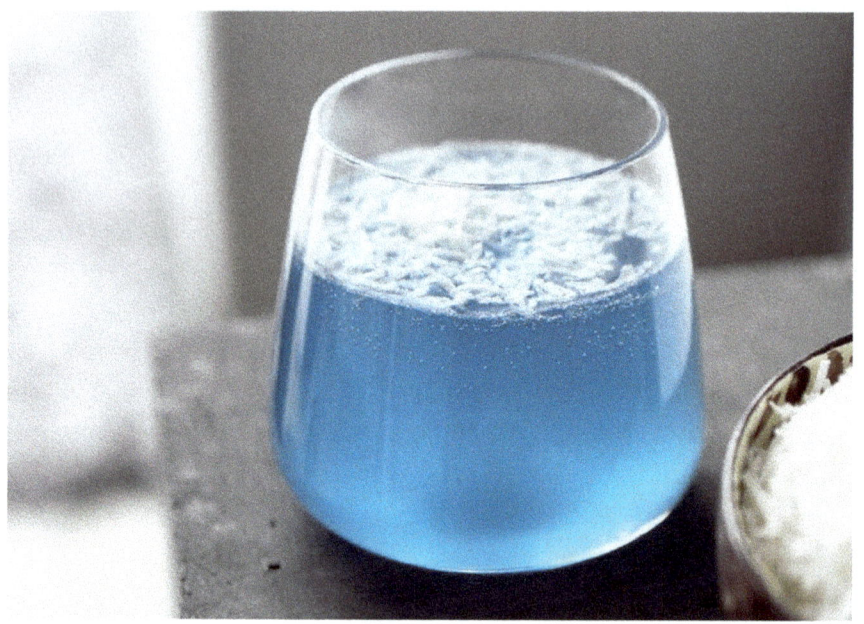

Makes: 1 serving

INGREDIENTS:
- 1-ounce coconut tequila
- ⅛ teaspoon spirulina powder
- Coconut water kefir
- Shredded coconut

INSTRUCTIONS:
a) In a cocktail glass, dissolve ⅛ teaspoon of spirulina powder with coconut tequila.
b) Add ice cubes and top with water kefir to your taste.
c) Stir gently and sprinkle with coconut shavings.
d) Serve immediately.

77. Açai Berry Spirulina Kombucha

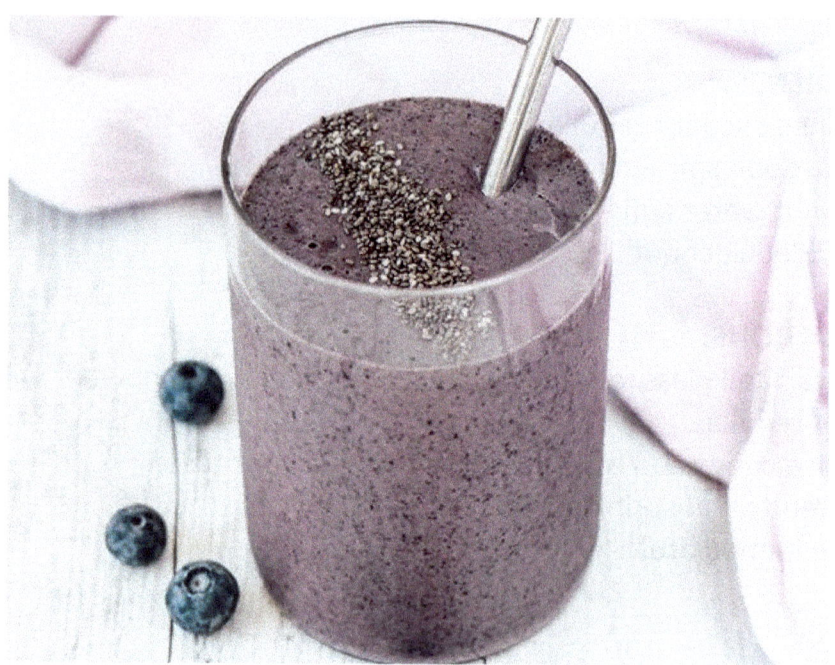

Makes: 1

INGREDIENTS:
- 4 ounces açai berry juice
- 4 ounces of black tea kombucha
- ½ teaspoon spirulina powder

INSTRUCTIONS:
a) In a glass, mix the juice, kombucha, and spirulina powder and serve.

78. Spirulina Yogurt Smoothie

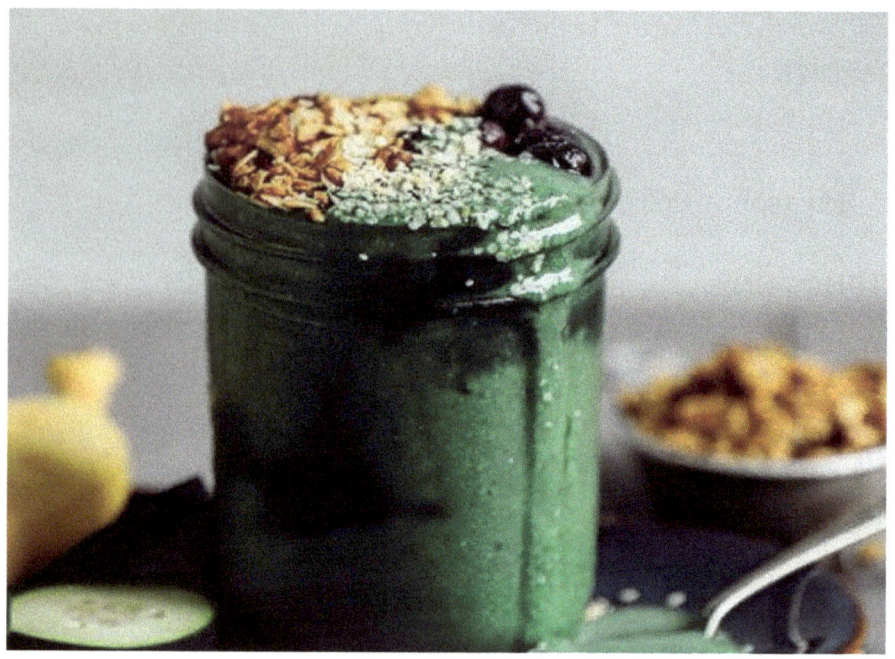

Makes: 2

INGREDIENTS:
- 1 teaspoon spirulina
- 2-3 centimeters ginger knob grated
- juice of ½ a lemon
- ½ cucumber
- A handful of spinach leaves
- 1 cup of yogurt
- ½ cup frozen blueberries
- ½ cup of water or more if needed

INSTRUCTIONS:

a) Blend the spirulina with the spinach leaves yogurt and some water.

b) Then add the cucumber, frozen blueberries, lemon juice, and ginger to the mixture, and blend thoroughly. Add more water if needed.

c) Garnish with some granola.

79. Protein Spirulina Limeade

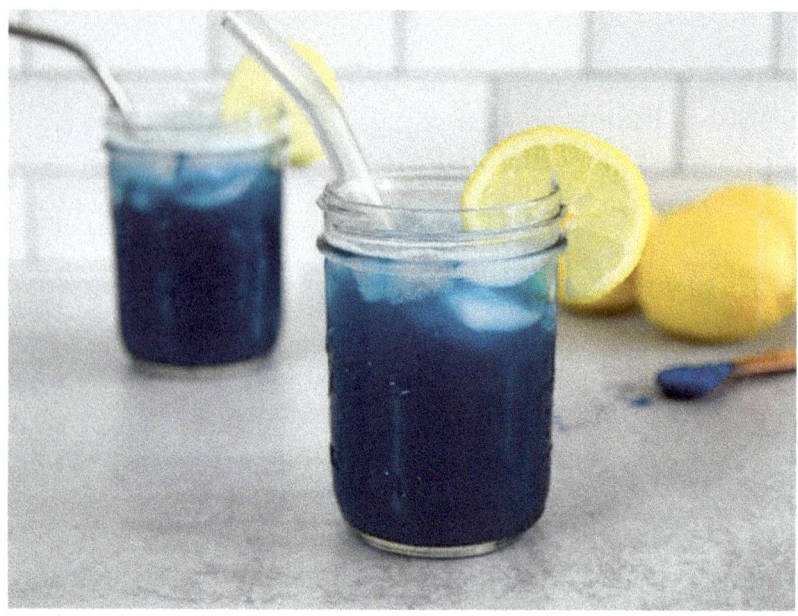

Makes: 2 Servings

INGREDIENTS:
- 1 apple
- 1 bunch watercress
- 1 lime, peeled
- 1 nectarine
- 1 pear
- 1 tablespoon spirulina powder

INSTRUCTIONS:
a) Simply put all the ingredients into your juicer.
b) Juice and serve in thoroughly chilled glasses.

80. Fruit And Cilantro Juice

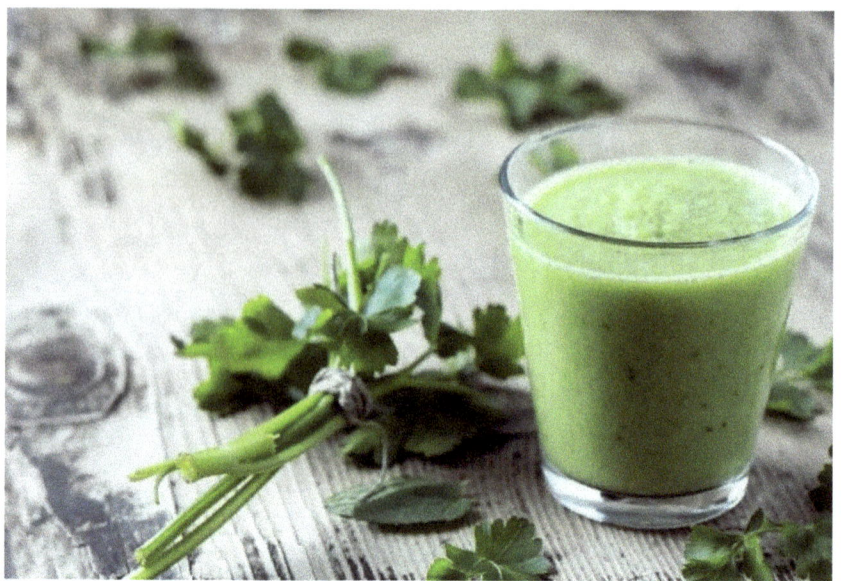

Makes: 2 Servings

INGREDIENTS:
- 1 bunch of fresh cilantro
- 1 lime, peeled
- 1 pear, cored
- 1 teaspoon Spirulina powder
- 2 Granny Smith apples, cored
- 4 stalks of celery, chopped

INSTRUCTIONS:
a) Juice celery, apples, pear, cilantro, lime, and spirulina in your electric juicer.
b) Split the juice between two tall thoroughly chilled glasses; serve immediately.

81. Cabbage And Orange Juice

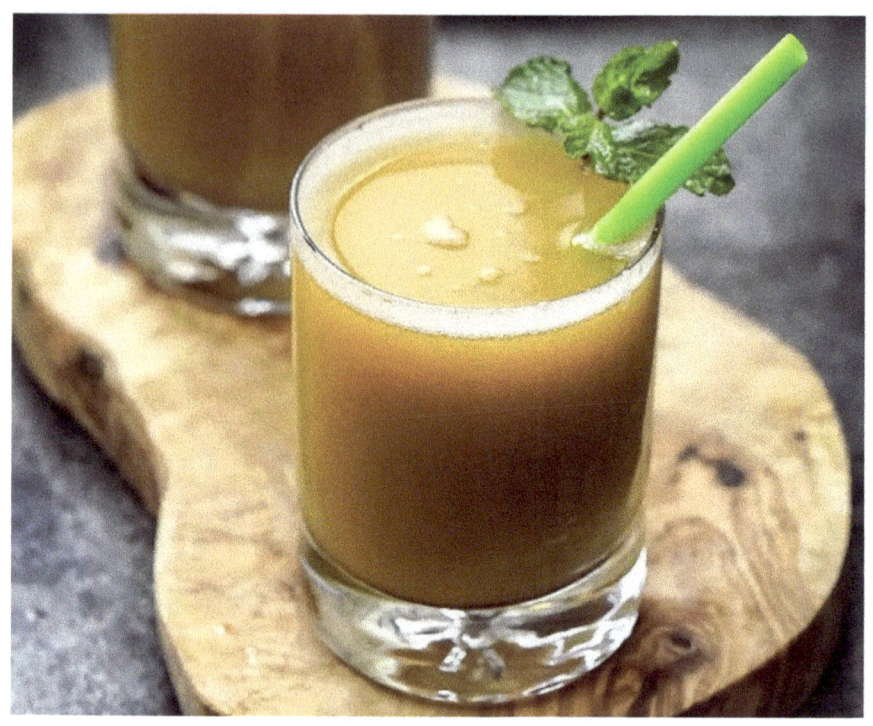

Makes: 2 Servings

INGREDIENTS:
- 1 green apple
- 1 orange
- 1 teaspoon Spirulina powder
- 4 leaves red cabbage

INSTRUCTIONS:
a) Core green apple and peel the orange.
b) Move them to a juicer together with cabbage and Spirulina powder.
c) Juice and serve immediately.

82. Papaya & Spirulina Smoothie

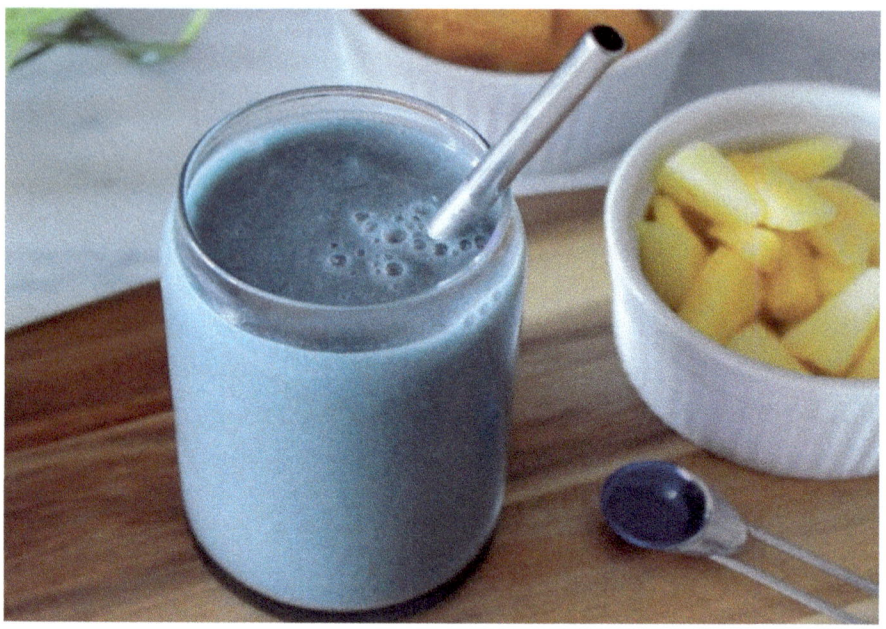

Makes: 2 servings

INGREDIENTS:
- 1 teaspoon of fresh Spirulina
- 1 fresh papaya
- 1 juice of Lime
- ½ teaspoon of cinnamon
- Ice

INSTRUCTIONS:
a) Mix all **INGREDIENTS:** in a blender until smooth.
b) You can also put Bananas or Strawberries. Enjoy!

83. Blackberry Virgin paloma

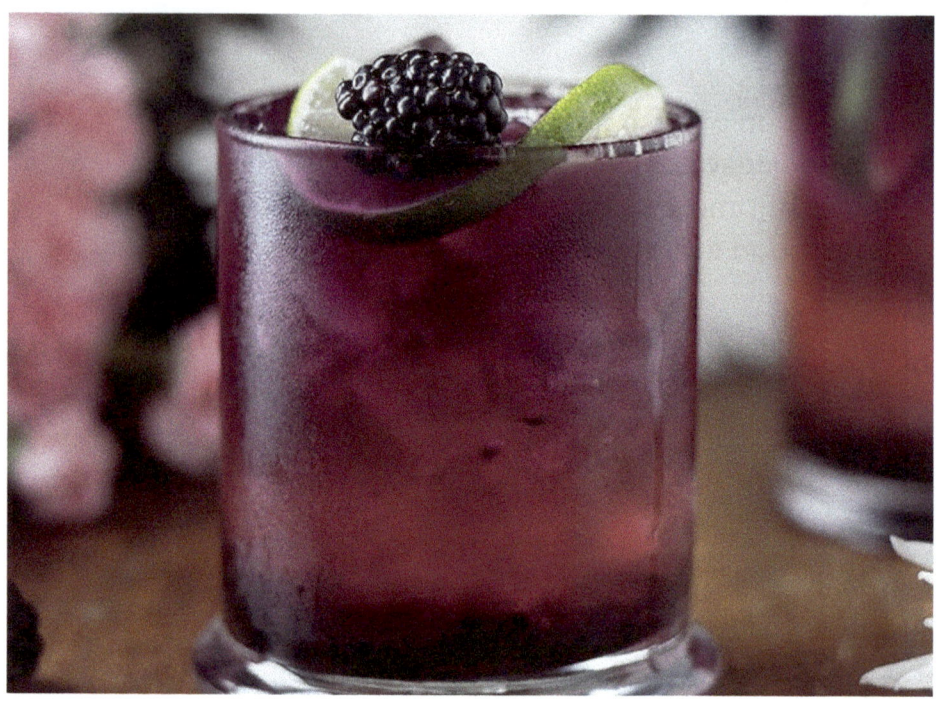

Makes: 1 Mocktail

INGREDIENTS:
- 3 Blackberries
- 5 dashes Hella Bitters Smoked Chili Bitters
- ½ ounce freshly squeezed lime juice
- 4-6 ounces of Grapefruit soda
- 1-ounce Spirulina tea, cooled

INSTRUCTIONS:
a) In a heavy-bottomed rocks glass, muddle blackberries. Add bitters and a squeeze of lime juice.
b) Top berries and bitters with a layer of crushed ice. This will keep the berry seeds from floating around in the drink.
c) Fill the glass with ice and top it with chilled grapefruit soda.
d) Add an ounce of cooled Spirulina for color, if desired. Garnish with lime and blackberries.

84. Spirulina Chamomile Kefir

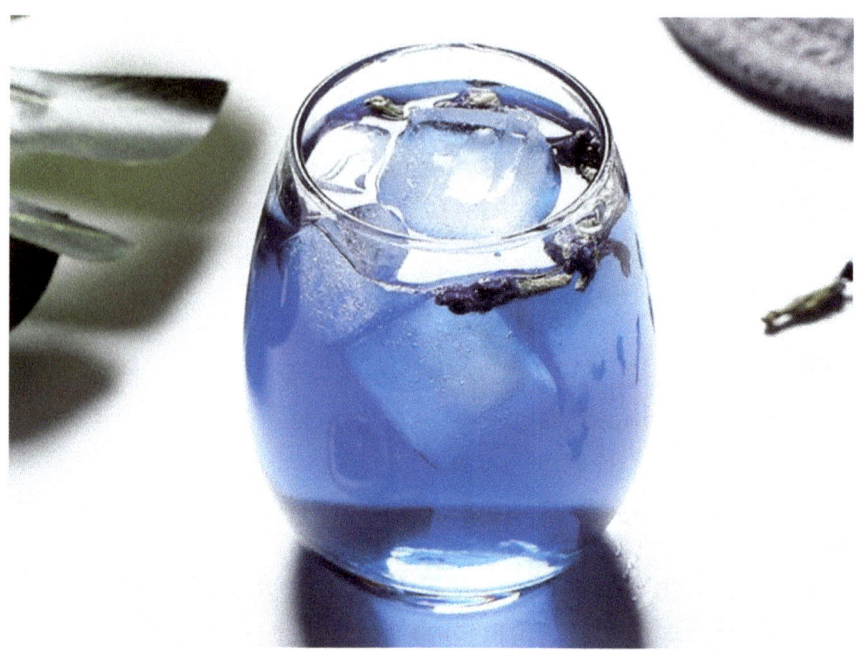

Makes: 4 cups

INGREDIENTS:
- 2 teaspoons spirulina powder
- 8 pieces of candied ginger
- 3 sprigs of fresh peppermint, bruised
- 1 teaspoon dried chamomile flowers

INSTRUCTIONS:
a) Make the first ferment and leave the jar in a warm place for 24-48 hours.
b) Strain the grains and add the ingredients to the green swivel top bottle with the first ferment water kefir.
c) Seal up the swivel top bottle and leave it in a warm place for 24 hours for the second ferment.
d) Open slowly, strain, and enjoy!

85. Spirulina Tea Latte

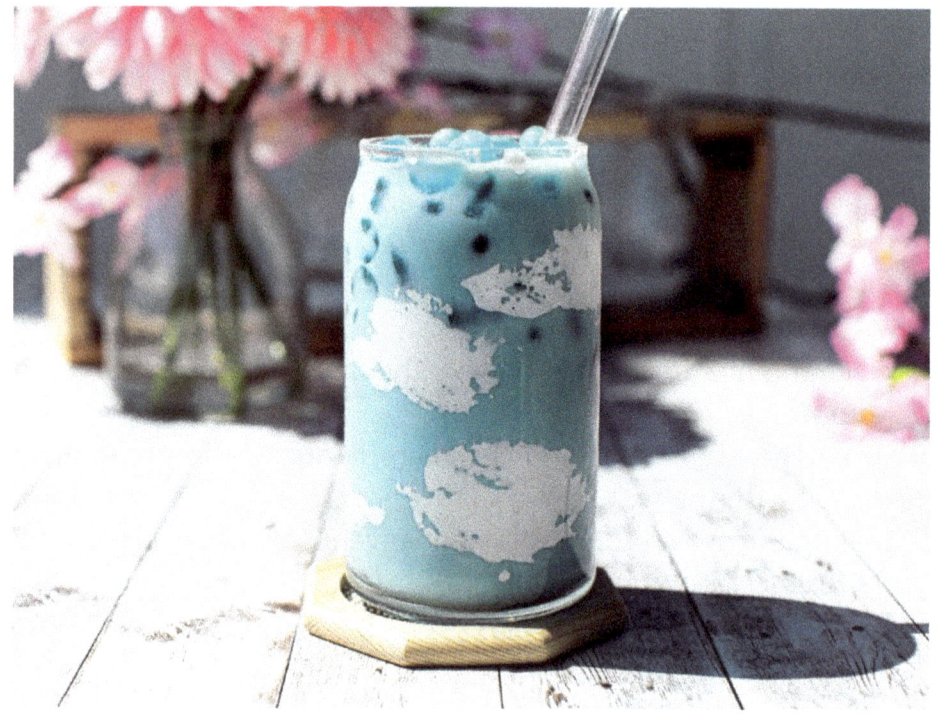

Makes: 4

INGREDIENTS:
- 1 teaspoon blue pea flower tea
- 8 ounces water
- ½ cup milk
- 1 teaspoon honey

INSTRUCTIONS:
a) Add loose tea leaves into an infuser.
b) Pour in a cup of hot water.
c) Allow steeping for 5 minutes. Don't overstep.
d) Steam the milk.
e) Pour the hot water into a mug.
f) Pour the milk on top.
g) Top with a drizzle of honey.

86. Green Coconut Berry Smoothie

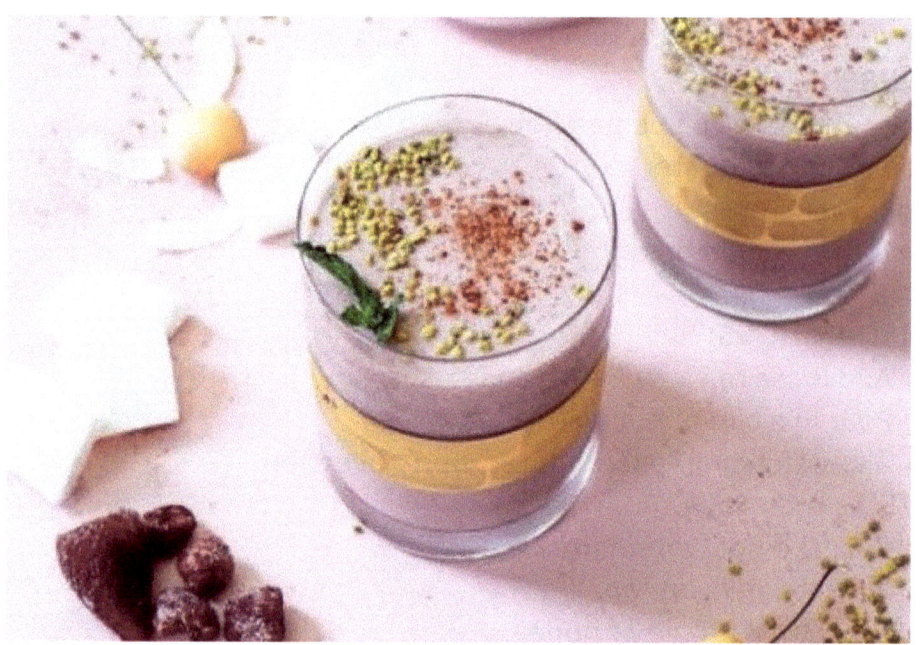

Makes: 2

INGREDIENTS:
- 1 cup fresh pineapple chunks
- 1 cup frozen blueberries
- 1 cup frozen mango chunks
- ½ cup of coconut water
- ¼ teaspoon Spirulina protein

INSTRUCTIONS:
a) Add all the ingredients and blend until smooth.
b) Garnish with chia and shredded coconut.

87. Papaya & Spirulina Smoothie

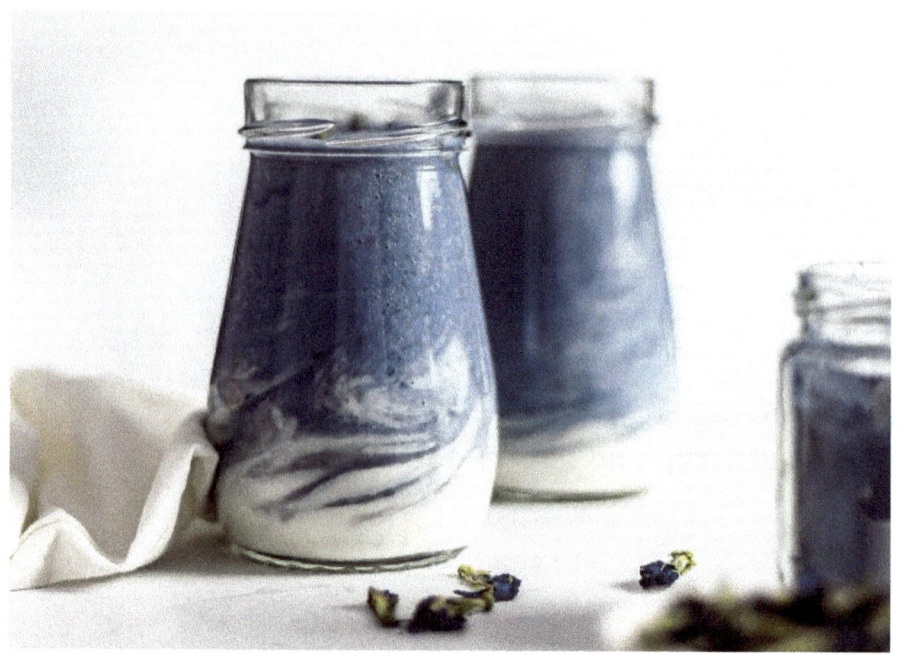

Makes: 2 servings

INGREDIENTS:
- 1 teaspoon of Spirulina powder
- 1 fresh papaya
- 1 juice of Lime
- ½ teaspoon of cinnamon
- Ice

INSTRUCTIONS:
c) Mix all ingredients in a blender until smooth.
d) Enjoy!

88. Spirulina Avocado Smoothie

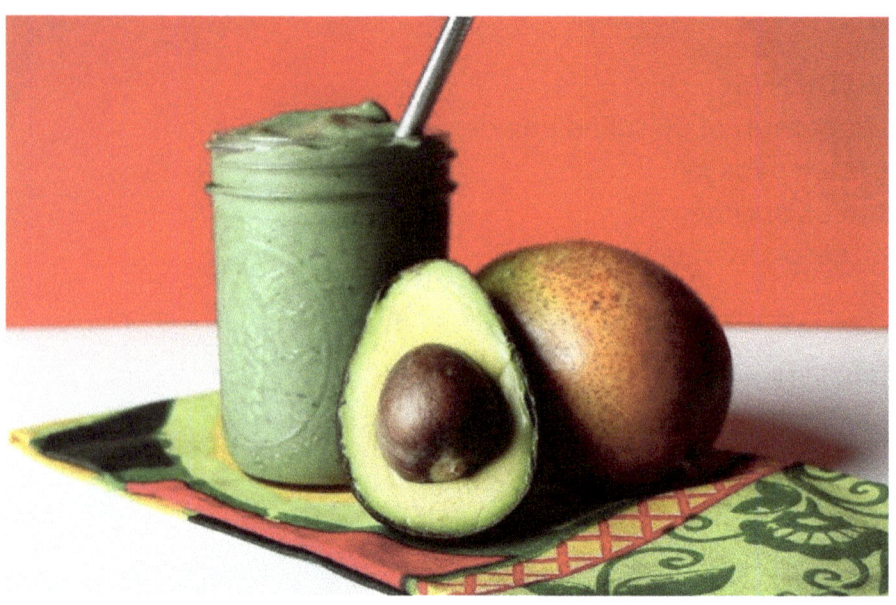

Makes: 3

INGREDIENTS:
- ½ avocado, peeled and cubed
- ⅓ cucumber
- 2 cups spinach
- 1 cup coconut milk
- 1 cup almond milk
- 1 teaspoon Spirulina powder
- ½ lime juice
- ½ scoop vanilla protein powder
- ½ teaspoons chia seeds

INSTRUCTIONS:
a) Blend avocado flesh with cucumber and the rest of the ingredients in a blender until smooth.
b) Serve.

89. Leeks Spirulina Smoothie

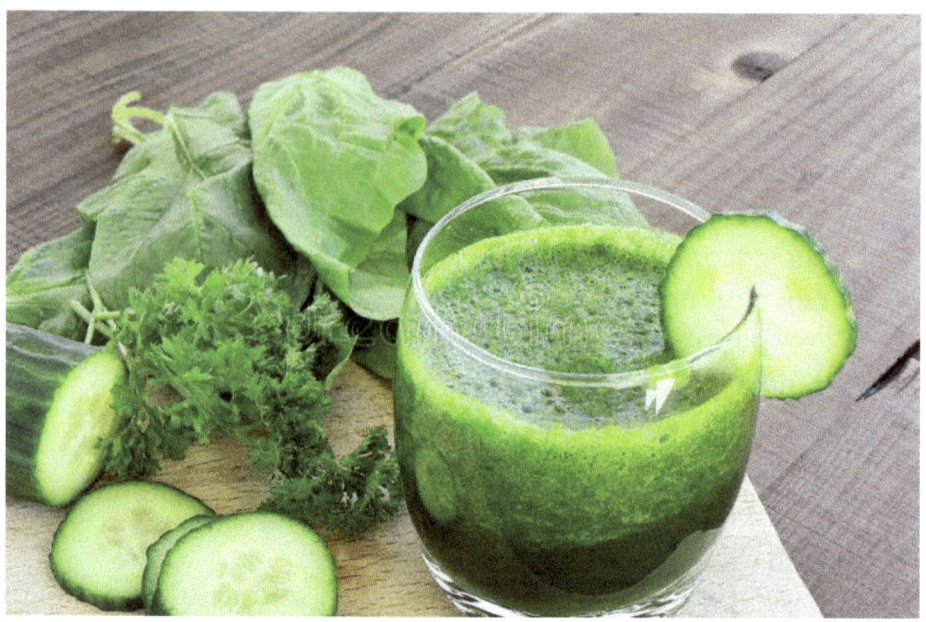

Makes: 2

INGREDIENTS:
- 1 cup Broccoli
- 2 Tablespoons Cashew butter
- 2 Leeks
- 2 Cucumbers
- 1 Lime
- ½ cup Lettuce
- ½ cup Leaf Lettuce
- 1 Tablespoons Spirulina
- 1 cup crushed ice

INSTRUCTIONS:
a) Combine in a blender.
b) Serve.

90. Cacao Spirulina Smoothie

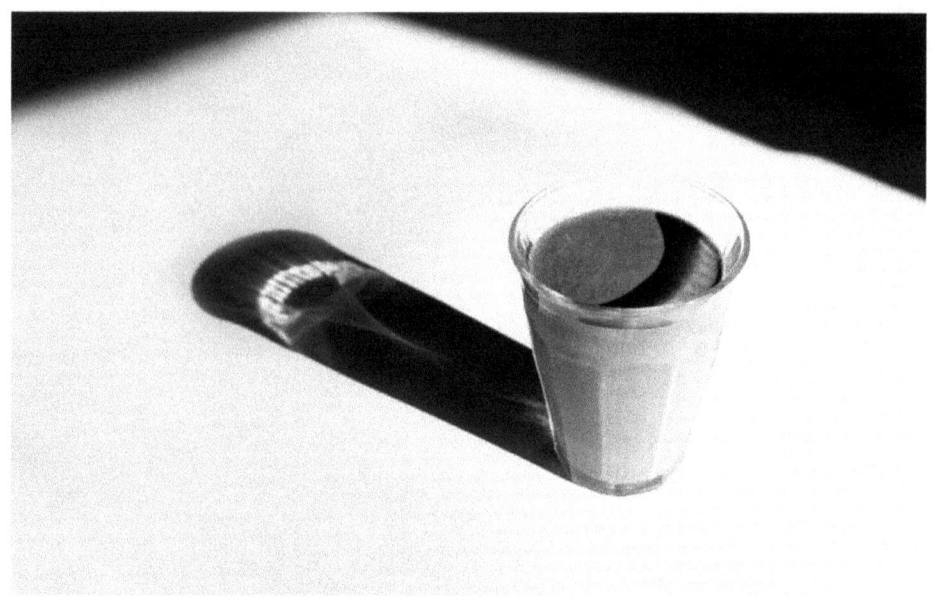

Makes: 2

INGREDIENTS:
- 2 cups spinach
- 1 cup blueberries, frozen
- 1 tablespoon dark cocoa powder
- ½ cup unsweetened almond milk
- ½ cup crushed ice
- 1 teaspoon honey
- 1 Tablespoons Spirulina powder

INSTRUCTIONS:
a) Combine in blender
b) Serve

91. Spirulina shake

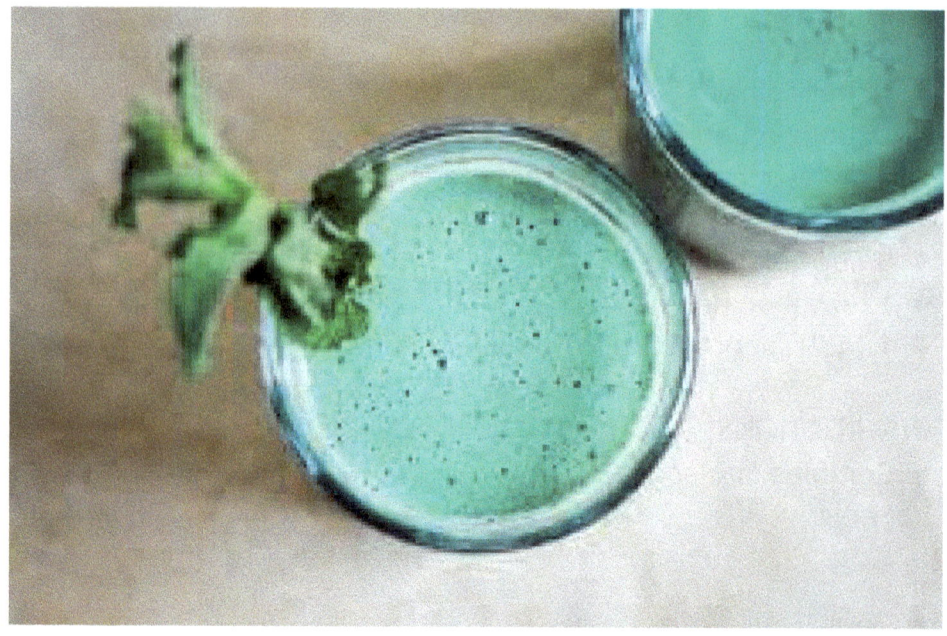

Makes: 4 servings

INGREDIENTS:
- ¾ cup almond
- ¾ cup pitted dates
- 1 tablespoon Spirulina
- 3 cups filtered water
- ½ teaspoon maca powder
- 1 cup ice

INSTRUCTIONS:
a) Combine the almonds, dates, Spirulina, water, maca, and ice in your high-speed blender and blend until smooth. Add the ice and blend until mixed well.

b) Best served immediately but will keep for several days in the fridge.

92. Spirulina & Ginger Smoothie

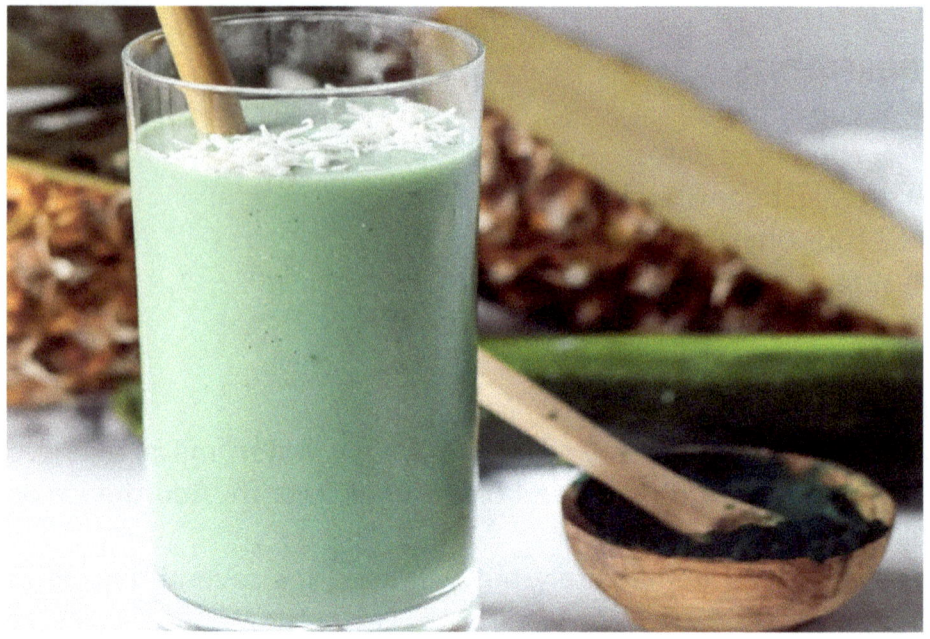

Makes: 2

INGREDIENTS:
- 1 Anjou pear, chopped
- ¼ cup white raisins or dried mulberries
- 1 teaspoon freshly minced gingerroot
- 1 large handful of chopped romaine lettuce
- 1 tablespoon hemp seeds
- 1 cup unsweetened Spirulina tea, cooled
- 7 to 9 ice cubes

INSTRUCTIONS:
a) Place all the ingredients except the ice in a Vitamix, and process until smooth and creamy.
b) Add the ice and process again. Drink chilled.

93. Spirulina Limeade

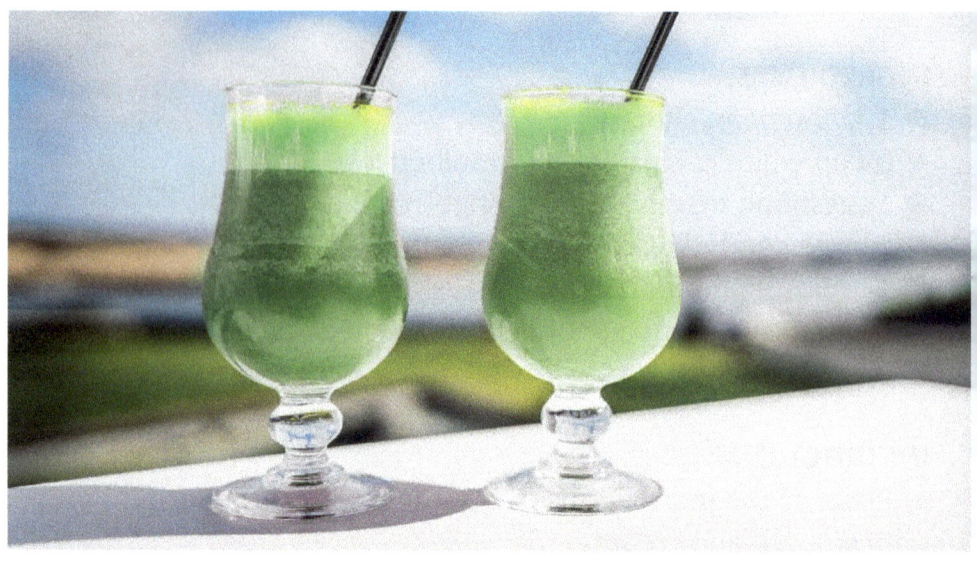

Makes: 20 servings

INGREDIENTS:
- 2 cups boiling water
- 1 tablespoon Spirulina powder
- 2 12-ounces cans of frozen limeade concentrate
- Garnish: lime wedges

INSTRUCTIONS:
a) In a teapot, combine boiling water and spirulina.
b) Let stand for 10 minutes.
c) Let the tea cool slightly.
d) In a large pitcher, prepare frozen limeade according to package instructions.
e) Stir in spirulina tea; cover and chill. Garnish with lime wedges.
f) Save the red juice from jars of maraschino cherries. Stir a little of it into the punch, lemonade, ginger ale, or milk for a sweet pink drink that kids will love.

94. Mint Chocolate Chip Shake

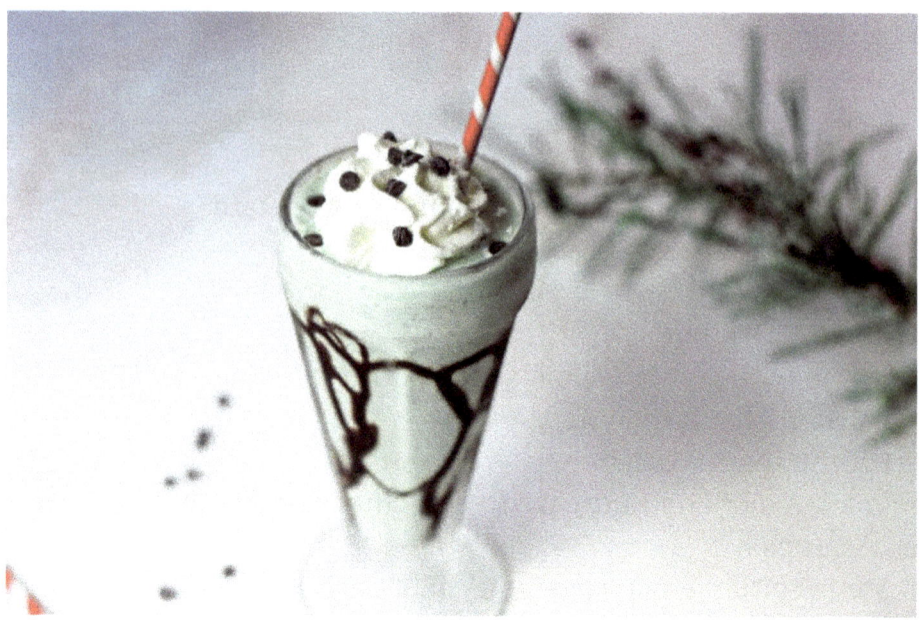

Makes: 2

INGREDIENTS:
- 2 scoops chocolate protein powder
- 12 ounces mint flavored Spirulina
- 1 Tablespoon raw cocoa powder
- 1 Tablespoon cacao nibs
- 3 Ice Cubes

INSTRUCTIONS:
a) Throw all ingredients into a blender for 30-60 seconds.

95. Vanilla Spirulina Avocado Shake

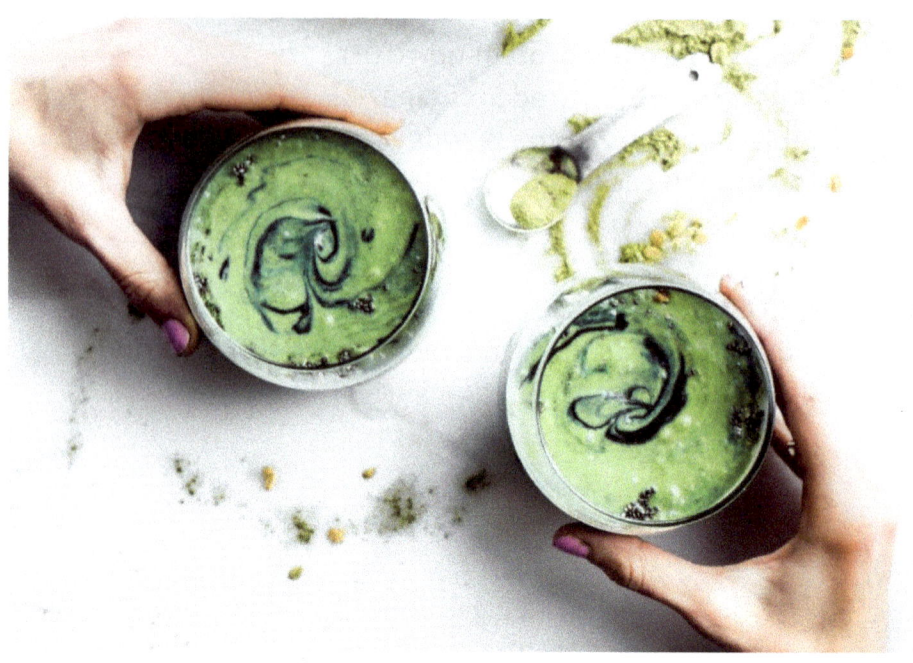

Makes: 2

INGREDIENTS:
- 1½ cups almond milk
- 2 scoops vanilla protein powder
- ¼ teaspoon vanilla extract
- ½ an avocado pitted and peeled
- 2 teaspoons Spirulina powder
- 1 handful of spinach

INSTRUCTIONS:
a) Blend until smooth.
b) Taste and adjust ice or ingredients if needed.

96. Spirulina And Coconut Frappe

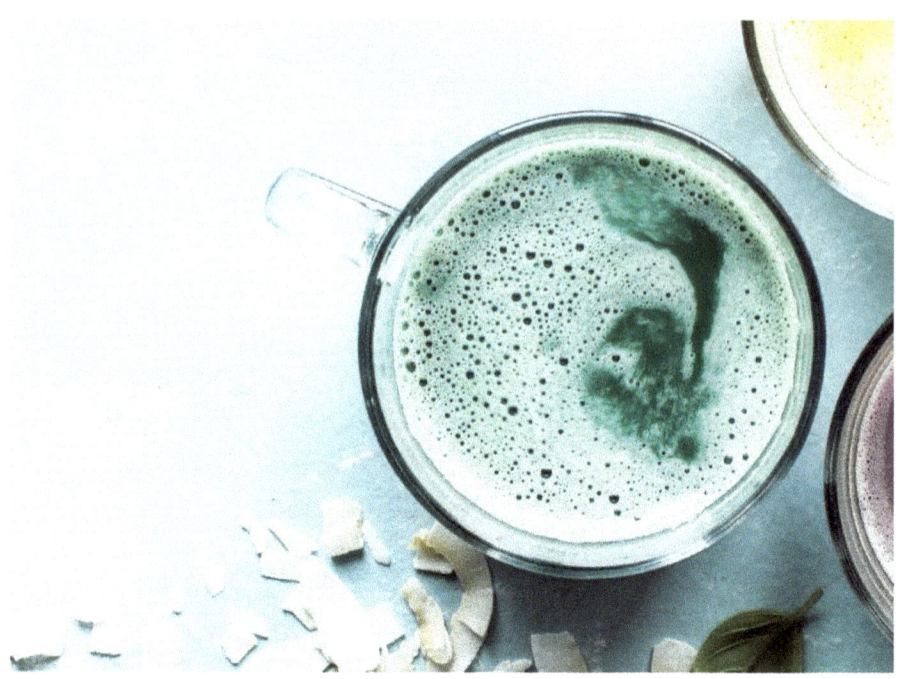

Makes: 2

INGREDIENTS:
- Ice + coconut milk
- 1 Scoop Yogurt frappé
- 1 mini scoop of Spirulina powder

INSTRUCTIONS:
a) Fill the cup with ice, level with the top of the cup
b) Pour milk over the ice
c) Pour the contents of the cup into a blender jug
d) Add frappé and Spirulina
e) Put the lid on tightly then blend until smooth

97. Spirulina & Strawberry Frappé

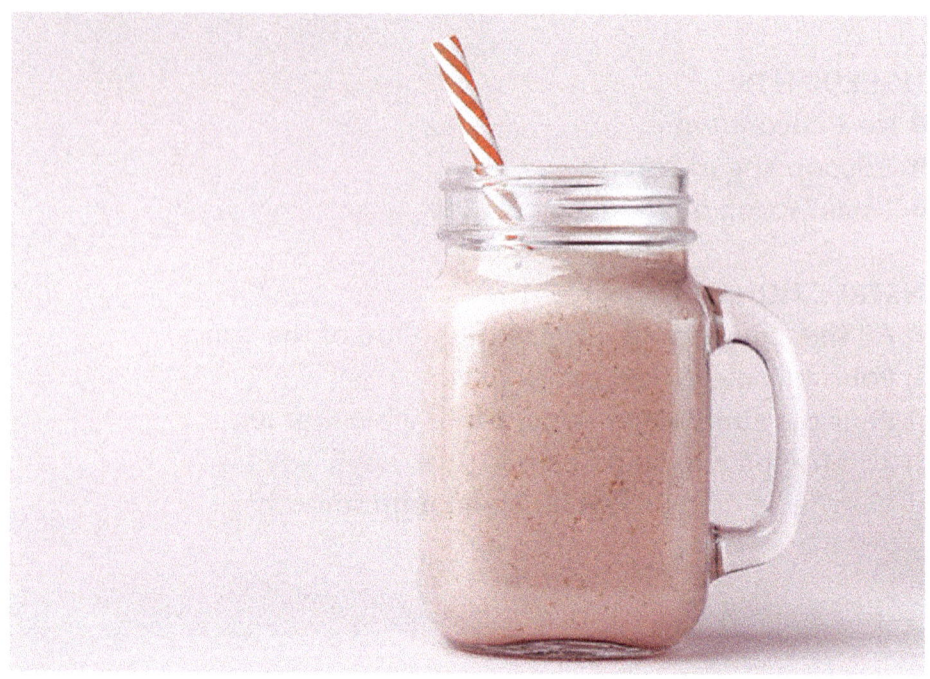

Makes: 2

INGREDIENTS:
- Ice + milk
- 1 mini scoop of Spirulina powder
- 2 pumps of Sugar-free Strawberry syrup
- 1 scoop White Chocolate frappé

INSTRUCTIONS:
a) Fill the cup with ice, level to the top of the cup
b) Pour milk over the ice
c) Pour the contents of the cup into a blender jug
d) Add Spirulina, syrup, and frappé powder
e) Blend until smooth

98. Spirulina Yogurt Smoothie

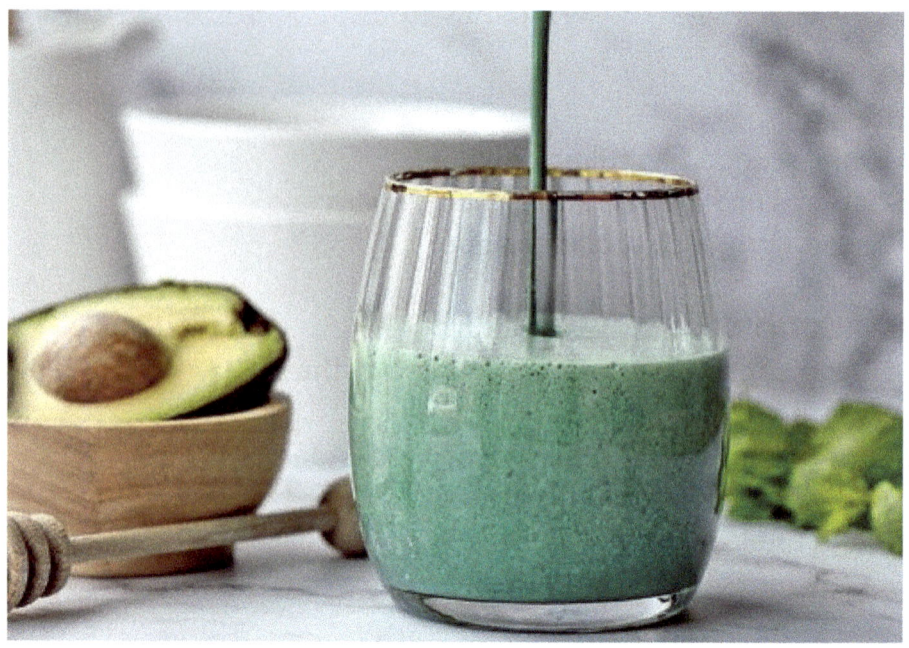

Makes: 2

INGREDIENTS:
- ½ cup of yogurt
- 2 tablespoons of honey or sugar
- ½ cup of ice cubes
- 1 teaspoon of Spirulina

INSTRUCTIONS:
a) Just put all the ingredients in the blender and mix them.

99. Spirulina Fruit Smoothie

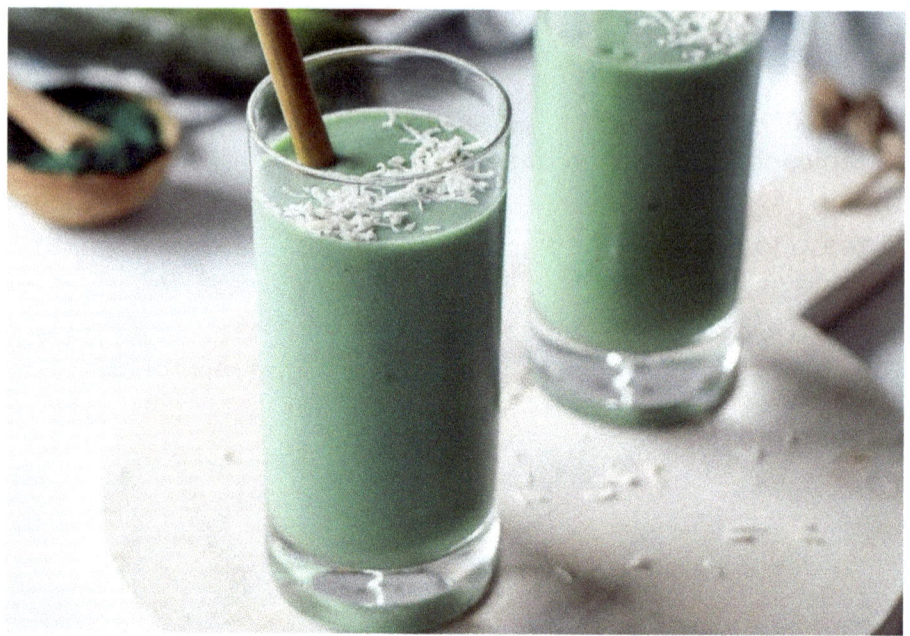

Makes: 2

INGREDIENTS:
- ¼ a cup of berries
- ½ cup of yogurt
- ½ cup of ice cubes
- 1 teaspoon of Spirulina

INSTRUCTIONS:
a) Blend ingredients in an electric blender and then pour the mixture into a tall class. It is preferable to drink it immediately after preparation.
b) You can add kiwis, bananas, mangos, and flavors of mint or ginger, it is all up to you and your preferences.

100. Blue-green Spirulina Milk

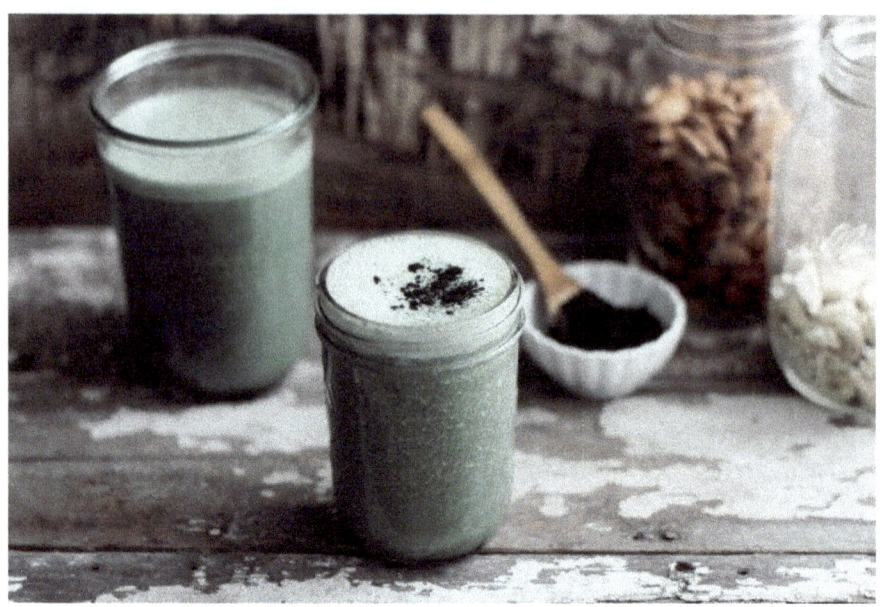

Makes: 4 servings

INGREDIENTS:
- 2 tablespoons spirulina, organic and powdered
- 2 cups filtered water
- ½ cup raw cashews
- ½ cup raw almonds
- 3 pitted dates
- ½ teaspoon vanilla extract
- pinch of sea salt

INSTRUCTIONS:
c) Soak the cashews and almonds for at least 2 hours in the water, and discard the water after soaking.
d) Blend all the ingredients in a blender until smooth. Chill before enjoying.
e) Keeps for 2-3 days in the fridge.

CONCLUSION

The Spirulina Cookbook is a must-have for anyone who wants to improve their health and energy levels with the power of spirulina. With its easy-to-follow recipes and comprehensive information on this superfood, this cookbook will help you make the most of this nutrient-packed ingredient in your daily life. Whether you're a health-conscious cook or just looking for some delicious new recipes to try, this cookbook is sure to become a staple in your kitchen.

These fun, bright-colored, and delicious spirulina recipes are simply magical! But spirulina is more than just a fun way to add visual excitement to your dishes. It has a ton of health benefits, too. Spirulina is packed with nutrients, it's anti-inflammatory, it can lower blood pressure, and so much more.

Now, spirulina on its own is more of an acquired taste. But don't worry, it's pretty easy to mask its flavor and these recipes are the best way to get started with spirulina.

Ingram Content Group UK Ltd.
Milton Keynes UK
UKHW020625210623
423802UK00010B/67